Dyslexia
A Beginner's Guide

Nicola Brunswick

ONEWORLD

OXFORD

A Oneworld Paperback Original

Published by Oneworld Publications 2009

Reprinted in 2012

Copyright © Nicola Brunswick 2009

The right of Nicola Brunswick to be identified as the
Author of this work has been asserted by her in accordance
with the Copyright, Designs and Patents Act 1988

ISBN 978–1–85168–645–2

Typeset by Jayvee, Trivandrum, India
Cover design by Simon McFadden
Printed and bound in Great Britain by
TJ International, Padstow

Oneworld Publications
185 Banbury Road
Oxford OX2 7AR
England
www.oneworld-publications.com

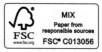

Learn more about Oneworld. Join our mailing list to
find out about our latest titles and special offers at:

www.oneworld-publications.com

For my mum and dad

Contents

Foreword

by Ken Follett, author and former President of Dyslexia Action

Let me guess: You know someone who might be dyslexic. It's your child, your brother or sister, or a colleague. And you're wondering if he or she can be helped.

Here's the good news: the answer is Yes. Most dyslexic people can learn to read and write normally.

The details are here in Dr Nicola Brunswick's informative book. She will tell you what dyslexia means, what we know about it, and – most importantly – what can be done.

Your dyslexic friend or relation can learn to read and write. It won't be easy. Dyslexics have to work harder than the rest of us to acquire these important skills.

They can't do it alone, either. Severely dyslexic people need special help. (Some mild dyslexics scrape by, especially if they're determined, but they do better with help.)

And your dyslexic acquaintance is already one of the lucky ones. Why? Because someone has noticed. That someone is you. And you have picked up a book about the problem. The worst thing that can happen to a dyslexic is that no one asks what's wrong. Most of them still go through life struggling to read and write and thinking – wrongly – that they're a bit stupid. It's a terrible waste of talent and causes much unnecessary suffering.

There are three dyslexics in my immediate family: two nephews and a stepdaughter. In their different ways they've all overcome the problem. They're grown up now. One is a lawyer, one is a doctor, and one runs his own business. It can be done! But you need expert guidance.

And this is a good place to start.

Preface

In 2003, the United Nations launched its Literacy Decade. Under the slogan 'Literacy as Freedom', its aim was to increase reading levels around the world, to improve individuals' chances of employment, increase their self-reliance, enhance their self-respect, and empower them to change their lives for the better.

Yet millions of people worldwide (around one in ten English-speakers) have dyslexia, a learning difficulty that seriously impairs their ability to read, write, and spell, find employment, and fulfil their potential. The fortunate ones are diagnosed early in their school lives and receive appropriate support and encouragement. They may progress to higher education and into employment. A recent study (described in chapter 8) has shown that around 35% of entrepreneurs in the United States are dyslexic. The unfortunate ones, whose reading difficulties are not identified or supported, may follow an altogether different path. Some estimates suggest that around 40% of prisoners are dyslexic.

Yet many myths abound regarding what dyslexia is and what it isn't. For example:

- Myth: Dyslexia is when people reverse letters, such as reading and writing a *b* as a *d*, and a *p* as a *q*.
- Truth: Some dyslexic readers reverse letters but so do many inexperienced non-dyslexic readers. This is not a typical symptom or cause of dyslexia.
- Myth: Dyslexia is when people are just a bit slow at reading.

- Truth: Slow reading is only one of the many signs and symptoms of dyslexia.
- Myth: Dyslexia is a phase that children grow out of.
- Truth: Dyslexia is a life-long condition.
- Myth: Dyslexic readers are not intelligent, and intelligent people cannot be dyslexic.
- Truth: Dyslexic people have average, or above average, intelligence.
- Myth: Given enough reading practice, dyslexic readers will eventually learn to read properly.
- Truth: Dyslexic people can use compensatory strategies to help them to read, but they will not overcome their dyslexia by reading practice alone.
- Myth: Dyslexia doesn't exist.
- Truth: It does.

This book is intended to dispel these and other myths about dyslexia, and to answer questions such as: are there different types of dyslexia? How is dyslexia diagnosed? When can the signs and symptoms of dyslexia be identified? Can anything be done to manage the difficulties of dyslexia? What is the most effective way of teaching dyslexic children? Does taking fish oil supplements help to alleviate the symptoms of dyslexia? Is dyslexia universal or does it occur only in speakers of alphabetic languages?

Readers who would like to know more about any particular topic are directed to the further reading suggested for each chapter, and to the other resources listed in the appendices.

At this point I'd like to thank a few people: my friend and colleague Dr Neil Martin for reading through earlier drafts of this manuscript, and for his ever-helpful advice on how to make it better; Marsha Filion at Oneworld, for commissioning me to write this book in the first place; and my husband, Jon, for his encouragement and support, and for making me many, many cups of tea while I wrote this book.

Nicola Brunswick, London

Illustrations

1

What is dyslexia?

> For me the toughest thing about dyslexia was learning to spell it.
>
> George Burns

What do you think unites the following people? Jamie Oliver, Michael Heseltine, Winston Churchill, Cher, Andy Warhol, Walt Disney, Hans Christian Anderson, Tom Cruise, Fred Astaire, Robin Williams, Tommy Hilfiger, John Lennon, Steve Redgrave, Richard Branson, Agatha Christie, Pablo Picasso. They have all achieved considerable success and fame in their chosen professions, true. They are all also, as you've probably guessed, dyslexic.

But what does this mean? The term dyslexia comes from the Greek *dys* – 'impaired' – and *lexis* – 'word', and refers to an impairment in the ability to read and spell that is not due to low intelligence or lack of educational opportunity. A number of different types of dyslexia has been identified. One general distinction is between acquired dyslexia and developmental dyslexia. We'll take a look at developmental dyslexia later in the chapter but start with a brief overview of acquired dyslexia.

Acquired dyslexia

Acquired dyslexia is a reading impairment resulting from brain injury (hence, the disorder is *acquired*). The most common forms of acquired dyslexia are deep dyslexia, surface dyslexia, and phonological dyslexia.

Deep dyslexia is a severe, but extremely rare, reading disorder where the patient experiences great difficulty reading simple words, such as *the, and, so,* and abstract words, such as *calm.* Nouns may be read although they will often be read incorrectly. For example, the word *sofa* might be read as 'soft', *dream* as 'sleep'. Made-up, nonsense words such as *grik* will not be read at all.

Surface dyslexia is a disorder in which patients are able to read regularly spelt real words such as *hand* and *mat,* and nonsense words such as *wolb,* but not irregular words such as *pint.* Regularly spelt words (or regular words) are pronounced according to the most common letter-sound patterns of the language, so *hand* is pronounced to rhyme with the similarly spelt words *land, stand* and *bland.* Irregularly spelt words (or irregular words) do not conform to common letter-sound patterns, so *pint* is not pronounced to rhyme with the similarly spelt (but regular) words *mint, glint* and *stint.*

Phonological dyslexia is an ability to read regular and irregular real words but an inability to read nonsense words. The term phonological refers to the speech sounds within language. A patient with phonological dyslexia, whose ability to appreciate the sound of language is impaired, is unable to convert the written letters of nonsense words (e.g. *filstromp*) into the sounds that they represent, so these words are not read.

Chapters 2 and 6 explore some of the explanations for these reading impairments. When the term dyslexia is used on its own, however, as in the title and contents of this book, it invariably refers not to acquired dyslexia but to *developmental* dyslexia.

Developmental dyslexia

Developmental dyslexia is an impairment in the *development* of skilled reading and spelling. Although there is no single, universally accepted, definition of developmental dyslexia, the many definitions that have been proposed generally describe its symptoms and hint at its possible cause; some also suggest ways in which its symptoms might be managed.

In one of the most widely cited definitions, the World Federation of Neurology (1968) suggests that developmental dyslexia is:

> a disorder manifested by difficulty in learning to read despite conventional instruction, adequate intelligence and socio-cultural opportunity. It is dependent upon fundamental cognitive disabilities which are frequently of constitutional origin.

Unfortunately, this prompts more questions than it answers. What is meant, for example, by 'conventional instruction'? What is 'adequate intelligence'? What is 'socio-cultural opportunity'? Which particular 'cognitive disabilities' distinguish a dyslexic reader from a poor reader? Little is revealed about the extent of the difficulties experienced, their possible cause or their effects. This definition suggests that dyslexia can only be identified *by exclusion* – i.e. people are only dyslexic if their reading difficulties cannot be explained by educational, intellectual or cultural factors. All this actually reveals is that children with reading impairments have unexplained 'difficulty in learning to read'.

The International Dyslexia Association (2002) has suggested a more advanced definition:

> Dyslexia is a specific learning disability that is neurological in origin. It is characterized by difficulties with accurate and/or fluent word recognition and by poor spelling and decoding abilities. These difficulties typically result from a deficit in the phonological component of language that is often unexpected in relation to other cognitive abilities and the provision of

effective classroom instruction. Secondary consequences may include problems in reading comprehension and reduced reading experience that can impede growth of vocabulary and background knowledge.

But again, this definition does not explain what dyslexia is or what causes it. For example, what is meant by the phrase 'neurological in origin'? What are these poor 'decoding abilities'? What is the 'phonological component of language'? And what is 'effective' classroom instruction?

In an attempt to provide a clear and accessible description of dyslexia, the British Dyslexia Association (2007) has offered the following definition:

Dyslexia is a specific learning difficulty which mainly affects the development of literacy and language related skills. It is likely to be present at birth and to be lifelong in its effects. It is characterised by difficulties with phonological processing, rapid naming, working memory, processing speed, and the automatic development of skills that may not match up to an individual's other cognitive abilities. It tends to be resistant to conventional teaching methods, but its effects can be mitigated by appropriately specific intervention, including the application of information technology and supportive counselling.

Although this definition is not without its problems either – for example, if dyslexia 'mainly affects' language and literacy skills, what else does it also affect? If it is only '*likely* to be present at birth', is this not always the case? If it is not present at birth, then what causes it to develop later in life? What is an 'appropriately specific intervention'?

Laying these problems aside, these last two definitions together offer more objective criteria for the identification of dyslexia. They identify it as a collection of reading, spelling, naming, and memory impairments caused by problems with perceiving and manipulating the sounds of language, and with associating written letters with their spoken representations. Written letters that represent individual spoken sounds are called graphemes. The spoken sounds that these graphemes represent are called phonemes. So, converting written letters (e.g. *b* or *eigh*) into their corresponding sounds ('buh' and 'ay') is known as grapheme-phoneme conversion. Difficulties with phonological processing and grapheme-phoneme conversion lie at the heart of dyslexia.

Poor phonological processing skills and poor grapheme-phoneme conversion ability make dyslexic readers less able than non-dyslexic readers to:

- read words by breaking them down into their component letters, converting these letters into their spoken sounds and blending these sounds together into a single word;
- spell words by breaking spoken words down into their component sounds, converting these sounds into individual written letters or strings of letters and writing these letters as a single word;
- hold verbal information in short-term memory;
- learn sequences of things – e.g. months of the year or times tables;
- recognise and produce rhymes;
- recognise the same sound in groups of words, such as *sun, sea and sand*;
- name objects, colours, or numbers quickly and accurately;
- pronounce long words – e.g. *perpendicular*.

Together, these difficulties impair the development of reading and spelling accuracy, they reduce reading comprehension ability, limit vocabulary, and hinder verbal communication.

Signs and symptoms of dyslexia

The specific signs and symptoms of dyslexia are extremely variable and depend on the person's age, sex, family background, educational experience, level of intelligence, and whether they also have other developmental problems. That said, the presence of a large number of symptoms should persuade individuals, parents, teachers, and psychologists to be on the lookout for dyslexia. Bear in mind, however, that not all dyslexic readers will display all of the symptoms, and where symptoms are seen, they will not necessarily be displayed to the same degree. Some symptoms, of course, may also be seen in people who are not dyslexic.

Despite this variability, you might expect to see clusters of particular signs and symptoms of dyslexia at specific stages of development. Some of the more typical ones are listed over the next few pages.

Early signs of dyslexia in pre-school children

- delayed speech development, i.e. not speaking by the age of two to three years;
- persistent difficulties with the pronunciation of multi-syllabic words, e.g. *animal* might be pronounced as 'aminal', *hospital* as 'hopital';
- difficulty learning nursery rhymes, and providing rhymes for simple words such as *cat* or *door*;
- difficulty learning spoken letter/word sequences, e.g. days of the week, the alphabet, or numbers;
- difficulty playing simple sound games, e.g. 'I spy with my little eye';
- difficulty acquiring new vocabulary, even familiar words, e.g. *table* or *milk*;
- showing no particular interest in written letters and words;
- difficulty clapping out a fairly simple rhythm;

- difficulties getting dressed – putting clothes on properly, and in the correct order – and putting the correct shoe on the correct foot;
- difficulty following simple spoken directions, particularly if two or more instructions are involved;
- problems with catching, kicking, or throwing a ball.

Signs of dyslexia in primary school children (five to eleven years)

- attempts to avoid reading out loud;
- reading that is hesitant and laboured – the child may become tired quickly;
- difficulty sounding-out unknown words;
- frequent loss of place in the text when reading;
- the same word read correctly and incorrectly in the same piece of writing;
- frequent omission and/or repetition of words when reading;
- inaccuracy in reading similar-looking words, e.g. *saw* and *was*, *lots* and *lost*;
- poor reading comprehension;
- a significant difference between written and spoken language ability – e.g. written work that is poorer than would be suggested by a child's spoken answers in class;
- messy handwriting, including much crossing-out;
- effortful-looking handwriting;
- frequent misspellings, even of high-frequency (common) words;
- bizarre spelling resulting from confusion between letters, e.g. writing *p* as *q*, *m* as *w*, *f* as *t*;
- the same word spelt differently in the same piece of writing, e.g. *catch* and *cach*;
- continued difficulty with pronouncing multi-syllabic words such as *microscope*;

- taking much longer than expected to complete written work;
- memory limitations, e.g. difficulty remembering months of the year, multiplication tables, classroom instructions;
- short attention span – the child is easily distracted from his/her work;
- frequent confusion between left and right, and a generally poor sense of direction;
- clumsiness;
- frustration, which may lead to behavioural problems in the classroom;
- poor confidence.

Signs of dyslexia in secondary school children (twelve to sixteen years)

Many of the reading, writing, and spelling problems of primary school-age children will still be seen in secondary school-age children. The following signs can also be found:

- written work containing many spelling mistakes that should easily have been identified and corrected;
- poorly planned, poorly structured written work that does not properly reflect the pupil's abilities;
- poor time-management skills leading to problems completing written work on time;
- difficulty taking written notes during class;
- classroom instructions need to be repeated;
- difficulty following the school timetable, and remembering which books to bring to class each day (symptomatic of poor memory and poor organisational skills);
- difficulty remembering mathematical formulae, poetry, and foreign language vocabulary;
- difficulty completing written tests and exams in a structured and coherent way;

- poor pronunciation of long words, such as *extraordinary* or *temporary*;
- low self-esteem.

Dyslexic readers, however, are frequently resourceful and develop compensatory strategies to help them to cope with, or even hide, these difficulties in the classroom. One rather extreme strategy is described below:

> Daniel, aged 12, knows that the class will be asked to real aloud … at 10 o'clock in the morning. At 9.45, he suddenly begins throwing balls of scrunched-up paper across the room at a class-mate. It's just a matter of time before the teacher, Mrs Stein, notices his behaviour and sends him into the hall to sit on the bench. For now, Daniel has won. He's spared the experience of reading aloud in front of his classmates.
>
> *The Secret Life of the Dyslexic Child* by Robert Frank, p. 35

Other compensatory strategies might involve:

- tape-recording lessons to avoid the need to take contemporaneous written notes;
- using computers with spell checks and grammar checks;
- having other people read through written work to check for errors; and
- allowing a longer than expected time to complete written work.

The author, John Irving, used this last strategy at school, as he recalls:

> I would ask my friends, 'How long did the history assignment take you? How long did the English assignment take you?' And if they said, 'Oh, it's 45 minutes', I would just double the time, or triple the time, and I'd say, 'Well, it's an hour and a half for me'. I just knew that everything was going to take me longer.

These strategies do not alter the underlying difficulties of dyslexia but they can help to hide many of its effects. In turn, this can make dyslexia more difficult to detect.

Signs of dyslexia in adulthood

While dyslexia is often first diagnosed in childhood, it is a life-long difficulty. The following signs and symptoms are often characteristic of the adult dyslexic reader:

* poor spelling;
* poor time-management – often arriving late for appointments or missing them completely;
* difficulty with planning and organisation;
* difficulty following directions, with confusion between left and right;
* having a more menial occupation than expected, based on their level of intelligence;
* difficulty taking down messages, especially if these involve strings of numbers – e.g. telephone numbers;
* avoidance of reading and writing wherever possible.

Many dyslexic readers receive intensive reading instruction throughout childhood and they learn to compensate for their early reading difficulties, but other signs usually remain throughout life. Poor spelling, in particular, is a typical sign of dyslexia in adulthood. For example, Agatha Christie, one of the world's most successful authors, had this to say about her dyslexia:

> I, myself, was always recognised . . . as the 'slow one' in the family. It was quite true, and I knew it and accepted it. Writing and spelling were always terribly difficult for me. I was an extraordinarily bad speller and have remained so until this day.

Another excellent example of the spelling difficulties experienced by adult dyslexic readers comes from an article written by

Lynn Barber in the UK's *Guardian* newspaper (19 March 2000) about her first meeting with the severely dyslexic writer and restaurant critic, A.A. Gill:

> Is he really dyslexic, or just a bit bad at spelling? He presses a key on his computer to reveal the work in progress and I am properly silenced. I must have interviewed several dozen people who describe themselves as dyslexic (sometimes I think being dyslexic is the prime requirement for being famous), but I have never actually seen the scale of the problem before. Adrian's spelling is so bizarre the computer spell-check is useless because it can't guess what word he is aiming for.

You may experience the same feeling when you attempt to read some of the words in figure 1. These words were written by an intelligent twenty-year-old dyslexic university student. How many of the words are you able to identify?

RUN	INSITUTE
ARM	LITRITURE
TRAIN	REVERANCE
SHOUT	MUSEUM
CORECT	PRESHOUS
SURCUAL	ICOGICALE
HEVAN	DISIGEN
EDUCATE	QUANTETY
MATIRIAL	IGSEGITIVE
REWEN	NISESITY

Figure 1 The spelling of an adult dyslexic reader

In case you're not really sure, these words are:

RUN	INSTITUTE
ARM	LITERATURE
TRAIN	REVERANCE
SHOUT	MUSEUM
CORRECT	PRECIOUS
CIRCLE	ILLOGICAL
HEAVEN	DECISION
EDUCATE	QUANTITY
MATERIAL	EXECUTIVE
RUIN	NECESSITY

The enduring problems of dyslexia are also summed up in the following quotation from an educational psychologist who recalls his feelings, as an adult, on being asked to read aloud in front of a room full of his colleagues:

> I was amazed on that day to find the same sense of fear pulsing through my body that I had felt as an 8-year-old child being asked to read aloud in class. Even as an adult with a PhD, I take my learning disability everywhere, every day of my life. Each day, I must learn to deal with it again; dyslexia is a secret I carry with me wherever I go.
>
> *The Secret Life of the Dyslexic Child* by Robert Frank, p. 21

Are there sub-types of dyslexia?

As the number and extent of signs and symptoms is so variable, it is often helpful to have a shorthand way of classifying individuals with common dyslexic difficulties, i.e. to identify sub-types of developmental dyslexia. Two main types have been distinguished – phonological dyslexia and surface dyslexia:

- Phonological developmental dyslexia (similar to phonological acquired dyslexia) is characterised by a difficulty in converting written letters into their corresponding sounds. Individuals have difficulty reading unfamiliar real words and nonsense, made-up, words (e.g. *glomp*).
- Surface developmental dyslexia (similar to surface acquired dyslexia) is characterised by difficulty in recognising words visually, as whole units. Individuals have difficulty reading irregular words (e.g. *aisle* or *chord*).

A third sub-type – mixed developmental dyslexia – may exist where individuals have difficulty both recognising words as whole units and converting individual written letters within words into their corresponding sounds. Individuals have difficulty reading unfamiliar words, nonsense words, and irregular words.

It is universally acknowledged that problems processing sounds is a consistent feature of developmental dyslexia. However, the purely visual difficulties of surface dyslexia are rarely seen in the absence of sound processing difficulties. The majority of dyslexic readers, therefore, can be classified as displaying a mix of difficulties.

A historical perspective

The first recorded use of the term *dyslexia* was by Rudolf Berlin, a German doctor writing in 1872. He described an adult patient who showed difficulties with reading following brain injury (as you've already seen, this would now be called *acquired dyslexia*). Some of the earliest reports of developmental dyslexia were made by the Scottish ophthalmologist James Hinshelwood and the English physician W. Pringle Morgan who described unexpected, but specific, reading difficulties in their patients. In articles published in *The Lancet* (in 1895) and *The British Medical Journal* (in

1896), Hinshelwood and Morgan described these reading difficulties as 'congenital word blindness', believing them to result
from disease of the visual system, specifically a region called the
left angular gyrus of the brain. This region lies between brain areas
responsible for the analysis of visual information and language, and
it is believed to be where visual information from printed text is
converted into its spoken representation.

Hinshelwood observed that a surprising number of intelligent children and adults were unable to read by sight. He
explained this in terms of their impaired visual memory for
letters, words, and figures. At about this time Morgan described
the case of a fourteen-year-old boy, Percy – 'a bright and intelligent boy' – who had been in education since the age of seven,
yet who experienced severe and specific difficulty learning to
read and spell. As Morgan noted:

> the greatest efforts have been made to teach him to read, but,
> in spite of this laborious and persistent training, he can only
> with difficulty spell out words of one syllable.

Again this difficulty was explained in terms of impaired visual
memories, as Morgan suggested:

> [Percy] seems to have no power of preserving and storing up
> the visual impression produced by words – hence the words,
> though seen, have no significance for him. His visual memory
> for words is defective or absent.

This idea that developmental dyslexia was a problem with visual
perception was developed further, and famously, by the American
neurologist Samuel Orton. He noted that some children with
reading difficulties tended to reverse letters (e.g. *b* and *d*) and to
swap around the order of letters within words, so they would read
saw as 'was'. Orton named this phenomenon strephosymbolia
(from the Greek *strepho* – 'to turn' – and *symbolon* – 'a mark or
sign'). He believed that when we look at a printed letter or a

word, the side of the brain that is dominant for identifying the printed image (usually the left) analyses this letter or word as it is presented (i.e. in the correct orientation). At the same time, he thought that the other (non-dominant) side of the brain analyses the same letter or word in its reversed form, like a mirror image. While most people are able to suppress the reversed image of the non-dominant hemisphere, Orton suggested that a minority experience confusion between the two images. This confusion was believed to explain the reading and spelling errors – particularly letter substitutions and reversals – made by poor readers.

We now know that Orton's explanation for dyslexia – as well as the explanations suggested by Morgan and Hinshelwood before him – was essentially incorrect. There is no reason to believe that the non-dominant side of the brain analyses letters and words in their reversed form, and letter reversals are just one of many errors that dyslexic readers may make when reading and writing. Nevertheless, it is remarkable just how important the work of these men was in raising awareness of developmental dyslexia and in laying the foundations of research into its manifestation and causes. Their findings were important in drawing a link between the observed reading difficulties of dyslexia and abnormalities in the brain.

What is also remarkable is that the brain region identified by Hinshelwood and Morgan in the nineteenth century as underlying the reading problems of 'word blindness' (the angular gyrus), is a region now shown by twenty-first-century brain imaging studies to show abnormal brain activity in dyslexic readers. This is explored in more detail in chapter 6.

The identification of dyslexia

An estimated 5–15% of speakers of alphabetic languages will be diagnosed with dyslexia. Alphabetic languages, such as English,

French, Greek, Spanish, and Arabic, are those in which individual sounds are represented by letters of the alphabet. Given this incidence, that is over twenty-four million people in the US alone. Although some research suggests that dyslexia is more common in boys than in girls by a ratio of between 2:1 and 4:1, other research has found no consistent evidence of sex differences.

The precise incidence of dyslexia is unknown because dyslexic readers differ in the severity of their reading difficulties just as non-dyslexic readers differ in their reading abilities. This leads to regular debate amongst psychologists about where the cut-off line should be drawn between people who are simply poor readers, whose reading difficulties are the result of low intelligence, brain injury, lack of motivation, emotional immaturity, adverse social or educational conditions, and those whose enduring reading difficulties cannot be explained by any of these.

There are no blood tests or DNA tests for dyslexia, and x-rays and MRI scans will reveal nothing that is diagnostically useful (chapter 6 has an overview of brain imaging studies of dyslexia). Dyslexia can only be identified on the basis of someone's performance on a range of standardised tests of cognitive ability, of which a reading test is only one. Not all dyslexic readers will display the same results on these tests. Depending on factors such as age, educational experience, interests, and personality, they will not all report the same problems that their dyslexia causes in their daily lives, either. The importance of producing a clear and concise description of what dyslexia is and how it may be identified, therefore, cannot be over-emphasised.

Associated difficulties

Although developmental dyslexia is a *specific* learning difficulty, in around 30% of cases it occurs alongside at least one other developmental disorder. The characteristics of these disorders might include:

- impaired motor skills, balance, and coordination (dyspraxia/developmental coordination disorder – DCD);
- poor hand-eye coordination, slow and messy handwriting, difficulty copying written text, and poor fine motor control of the hands (dysgraphia, although these symptoms might also reflect the fine motor difficulties of dyspraxia);
- poor concentration, inattention, impulsivity, and hyperactivity (attention deficit/hyperactivity disorder – ADHD);
- difficulty with counting, performing mental arithmetic, understanding and applying mathematical concepts (dyscalculia).

There are similarities between the symptoms of these disorders and dyslexia. For example, poor handwriting, difficulty remembering numbers, and problems with balance and coordination. However, the extent to which any symptom or combination of symptoms is displayed will vary person by person. Therefore, it is vital that a dyslexia assessment is undertaken by a psychologist or a specialist dyslexia teacher who is aware of the commonalities and differences between these disorders.

A word about intelligence

Whatever the differences between the various definitions of dyslexia, one factor on which they all agree is that reading difficulties occur despite the person having average, or above average, intelligence. Phrases such as 'despite adequate intelligence' and 'difficulties … that are unexpected in relation to an individual's other cognitive abilities' have appeared in almost every definition of dyslexia. Even Morgan (1896) recognised the importance of describing Percy as 'a bright and intelligent boy', pointing out that:

The schoolmaster who has taught him for some years says that he would be the smartest lad in the school if the instruction were entirely oral.

That dyslexia occurs in people with average, or above average, intelligence seems to be lost on many, however. In 2005, a headline in the UK's *Daily Mail* newspaper quoted an educational psychologist from Durham University as saying that, 'Dyslexia is "just a middle-class way to hide stupidity" ', before going on to say:

After years of working with parents, I have seen how they don't want their child to be considered lazy, thick or stupid. If they get called this medically diagnosed term, dyslexic, then it is a signal to all that it's not to do with intelligence ... There are all sorts of reasons why people don't read well but we can't determine why that is. Dyslexia, as a term, is becoming meaningless.

This statement is incorrect and highlights the stereotype of the dyslexic person as lazy and/or stupid. Take a look at the following statements made by four dyslexic readers:

1. 'I performed poorly at school, when I attended, that is, and was perceived as stupid because of my dyslexia.'
2. 'I was called "stupid" a lot by many lovely kids at school, and that makes you pretty determined to learn to read ... and figure out ways around it.'
3. 'As a child, I was called stupid and lazy ... My parents had no idea that I had a learning disability.'
4. 'When I was a kid they didn't call it dyslexia. They called it ... you know, you were slow, or you were retarded, or whatever.'

So, what do these show? They all reflect prejudice and lack of understanding of dyslexia. But these people were far from lazy or stupid. They were, respectively, Tommy Hilfiger, world famous fashion designer; Keira Knightley, award-winning actress who has starred in films including *Bend it Like Beckham*, *Pirates of the Caribbean*, and *Atonement*; Henry Winkler, actor and TV producer, famous for his roles in *Happy Days*, *Laverne and Shirley*, and *Arrested Development*; and Whoopi Goldberg, multi award-winning star of *Jumpin' Jack Flash*, *Sister Act*, and *Ghost*.

Dyslexia, as you will see throughout this book, is associated with both strengths and weaknesses. As chapter 8 shows, if dyslexic students are taught in a way that exploits their strengths rather than their weaknesses, academic and professional success is achievable.

2

How we learn to read and spell

> To learn to read is to light a fire; every syllable that is spelt out
> is a spark.
>
> Victor Hugo (1802–1885)

Before studying impaired reading we have to understand the
mechanics of how we read, and how we learn to read normally.
By the time children start school, most of them are able to
understand and speak between 1,500 and 3,500 words. Their
spoken language skills – their knowledge of the rules of the
language (syntax) and the meanings of words (semantics) – are
developing rapidly, and their vocabularies are increasing by
around five words a day. At this stage of development children
only lack the linguistic talents specifically associated with reading
and spelling. These include the ability to recognise individual
letters and words, and to understand the relationship between
letters and their corresponding sounds. These skills are only
learned as a result of explicit instruction and considerable effort.

The artificial and complex processes that underlie reading
have been described by psychologist Philip Gough as 'an unnat-
ural act' involving 'cryptanalysis or codebreaking'. These
processes involve the accurate integration of printed visual word
forms (orthography), spoken word sounds (phonology), and
word meanings (semantics). At the simplest level, we extract
visual features from written text and combine these into whole
letters. Individual letters are combined into whole words and

these are then 'looked up' in our mental store of familiar words and their meanings (our mental lexicon). The average adult reader is familiar with around 50,000 words. If the word exists in the mental lexicon, i.e. if we know it, then its meaning may be retrieved. The meanings of the individual words within a sentence can then be combined, and we understand the sentence.

Various models have been developed in an attempt to explain in simple terms how we acquire these fairly sophisticated skills, and how we go from being pre-reading, pre-spelling, children to confident, fluent, adult readers and spellers.

The Cognitive Developmental model

Models of reading and spelling generally suggest that literacy skills develop in a discrete sequence of stages, each of which must be passed through before the child progresses to the next. The Cognitive Developmental model, for example, suggests that learning to read involves four developmental stages.

Stage 1

The child learns to recognise a few words by sight without any reliance on alphabetic or phonological knowledge. Earliest words are likely to include ones that they see frequently in their story books and around the home, such as *the*, *and*, *me*, and the child's own name. If an unfamiliar word is seen in a sentence the child may guess at the word on the basis of its context, selecting from their store of familiar words, although the guessed word is likely to bear little visual resemblance to the actual word. Unfamiliar words presented out of context will not be identified correctly. Phonology plays no part in this initial stage of word recognition.

Stage 2

During this stage, in the first year of reading, the child's visual word-recognition system is expanding. If shown an unfamiliar word in isolation they may guess with a word that is visually similar to the actual word. For example, the guessed word and the actual word may share the same first letter, so *window* might be read as 'walk', or the words may share the same first and last letters, so *running* might be read as 'ring'. Children at this stage are able to read familiar words but their lack of knowledge regarding the relationship between the spoken and written forms of letters and words renders them unlikely to read unfamiliar words correctly.

Stage 3

By the age of seven most children start to become familiar with the rules of grapheme-phoneme (letter-sound) conversion and they begin to decode words grapheme by grapheme. However, a grapheme is not necessarily the same as a single letter, but could be a cluster of letters that corresponds to a single spoken sound. For example, the spoken 'b' sound in the word *bloom* is represented by one letter. The spoken 'th' sound in the word *thanks* is represented by two written letters. The spoken 'igh' sound in *light* is represented by three letters, while the 'eigh' sound in *sleigh* is represented by four letters. Exactly how young children break words down into their constituent graphemes instead of attempting to read letter-by-letter is as yet unknown.

Children also learn to recognise that the same patterns of letters (e.g. *eak*) appear in different words with shared sounds (e.g. *peak*, *leak*, and *beak*). The child will start to 'sound out' words although they may produce non-words and read irregular words as if they were regular. An example of this would be if the word *watch* was pronounced to rhyme with *catch*, *match*, and *latch*.

As words are decoded they enter the child's visual word-recognition system. Phonological decoding remains an option, especially if the reader encounters unfamiliar words. Only 20% of all English words are used frequently in spoken and written language – these include words such as *the*, *and*, *with*. The other 80% of words – such as *abhor*, *derange*, *slovenly* – are used infrequently (on average, less than once for every million words that we use). Words that we encounter frequently become so familiar to us that we are able to recognise them quickly as whole words. Words that we encounter infrequently, however, are not so familiar; when we encounter these words in print we must break them down into their component letters and use our grapheme-phoneme decoding skills to read them.

Stage 4

Children's phonological decoding ability has developed to a sophisticated level by this stage. They have learned that some rules of grapheme-phoneme conversion, even in a language such as English, are inviolable. The letter 'c', for example, is pronounced as a 'k' sound when followed by the letters 'a', 'o', or 'u' (as in *car*, *college*, and *cup*), but as an 's' sound when followed by an 'i', 'e', or 'y' (as in *city*, *celery*, and *cyborg*). Children at this stage are also aware that words sharing the same written letters may be pronounced in the same way. So, knowing how to read the familiar word *catch* may help a child to read the unfamiliar word *latch* (although, as we have seen with the word *watch* this strategy may still cause problems). This process, known as 'reading by analogy', will be explained in more detail later.

While this model provides a useful description of the general steps that children take in learning to read, it is problematic in various respects. When confronted by an unfamiliar word a child must be able to sub-divide the word into letters or strings of letters which correspond to spoken sounds, and then reassemble these sounds into a recognisable word. However, this description of the process of grapheme-phoneme conversion, particularly in a highly irregular language such as English, may be overly simplistic. A child attempting to read the previously unseen word *bat* on the basis of its letter–sound correspondences, for example, will produce a nonsense word approximating to 'buhatuh'. Similarly, a child attempting to read the word *together* by breaking it down into its component parts – 'to', 'get', 'her' – will also experience difficulty. So this model, as it stands, is too descriptive without explaining how children acquire the skills that they need at each stage of reading development. For example, it fails to explain how they learn to identify graphemes within words, how they learn the rules of grapheme-phoneme conversion, and how different reading strategies might be used in the reading of familiar and unfamiliar words.

The 'Three Stage' model

Taking into account the failings of the Cognitive Developmental model, another theory developed by Professor Uta Frith – the Three Stage model of reading – explains reading acquisition in terms of the range of strategies that children are able to use as their reading skills develop.

Stage 1

Children recognise words, such as familiar product logos, on the basis of their visual form. This stage is described as logographic because a written letter or symbol represents an entire word without giving any indication of its pronunciation, much like a logo.

Stage 2

At this stage children continue to recognise words visually but as they become increasingly familiar with the alphabet they also begin to apply simple grapheme-phoneme rules to help them to identify written words.

These stages are viewed as being essentially equivalent to the previous model's first three stages.

Stage 3

This stage involves the use of previously learned logographic and alphabetic skills as well as the recognition of larger strings of letters within words. Children who know how to pronounce the letter sequence 'ight', for example, can use this knowledge to enable them to read words such as *might, sight, knight, flight*, and *delight*. By recognising larger letter strings as whole units, the child's reading becomes faster and more efficient.

It is this third stage which discriminates between these two models. In the Cognitive Developmental model, the reading strategies in use at each stage replaced the strategies of the previous stage. In the Three Stage model new strategies do not replace those of previous stages, they are used *in addition* to them.

While these models are appealing in that they help us to gain a general understanding of the steps that children take in learning to read, they have attracted criticism for their rigid adherence to the concept that children learn to read by progressing through a series of discrete stages. It may be more prudent to see the acquisition of reading as a succession of overlapping processes rather than a sequence of discrete, identifiable stages.

The 'Four Phase' model

The Four Phase model (proposed by Professor Linnea Ehri) describes reading development as a series of 'phases' rather than 'stages'. While the word stage suggests a distinct change from one period of development to the next, the word phase is used in this model to suggest a period of development that is rather more fuzzy at the edges.

Phase 1

Children in the initial – *pre-alphabetic* – phase of reading development have no knowledge of the alphabet or of the rules of grapheme-phoneme correspondence. When words in the child's environment are recognised, this is done solely on the basis of salient visual cues. For example, children may look at a product logo – the name of their favourite breakfast cereal or a fast-food restaurant, and immediately identify the name associated with the logo – but this is not reading as we think of it. The product/brand name would not be recognised out of context. Researchers have shown that changing the text on such logos has no effect on pre-literate children's identification of the products. Children shown the words LOCA COLA or XEPSI printed in their familiar designs will read COCA COLA and PEPSI without noticing anything wrong with the text.

Phase 2

As children enter the second phase (called *partial alphabetic*) they are already able to recognise some written letters. First and last letters within words, being the most salient visually, are often the ones that children will use to help them to guess an unknown word's identity. For example, in the word *carpet* the child may recognise the letters *c* and *t* and guess that the word says 'cat'.

Phase 3

By the time children have progressed to the third – *full alphabetic* – phase they are becoming more accurate in their identification of letters and letter clusters and increasingly familiar with grapheme-phoneme correspondence rules. These skills may be used in the reading of unfamiliar words. Children are also starting to build up a 'sight vocabulary' of familiar words which they are likely to recognise as whole words rather than by grapheme-phoneme conversion.

Phase 4

The final phase of this model – the *consolidated alphabetic* phase – is similar to the third stage of the Three Stage model. In this phase individuals become familiar with increasingly large strings of letters within words. The ability to identify larger letter strings by sight reduces the memory load involved in reading and speeds up the reading process. A child who is familiar with the letter clusters 'qu', 'est', 'tion', and 'ing', for example, should have little difficulty quickly joining these together in their memory to read by sight the word *questioning*.

Unlike the previous models, this one does not suggest that children progress sequentially from one phase to the next. Instead, it recognises overlap between the skills that children use in different phases so it is able to describe, in general terms, the route that children follow as they learn to read. However, it is possible that some children bypass some phases. For example, research has shown that children with good early phonological skills do not pass through the pre-alphabetic/logographic phase of reading but go straight to the partial alphabetic phase. Some reading researchers have even criticised the inclusion of the pre-alphabetic phase in the model. They suggest that children's identification of words while they still have no knowledge of the alphabet is irrelevant to our understanding of alphabetic reading development. Others have criticised the model for explaining nothing about skilled reading. A child's reading of words by breaking them down into their constituent letter strings is not the same as an adult's reading of words as whole units.

Reading 'by analogy'

A common thread running through each of these models is the importance of understanding that words sharing common sounds also often share letter sequences. As children are taught to read they are shown how to break words up into their constituent parts. One way of doing this is to divide them at the point of the first vowel, so the consonants that precede the vowel are split from the vowel and its succeeding consonants. For example, with the word *string*, the 'str' would be split from the 'ing'. The technical terms for these components are the *onset* and the *rime*. Words can then be grouped together into word families based on a sharing of common onsets or rimes. Some examples are shown in Table 1.

Table 1 Some simple word families that share common onsets and rimes

A few members of the 'str-' onset family:	A few members of the '-ing' rime family:
• straw	• bring
• stray	• cling
• stream	• fling
• street	• king
• string	• ping
• stripe	• ring
• stroke	• sting
• strong	• swing
• struck	• thing
• strut	• wing

English has thirty-seven rimes, including -ack, -ail, -ing, -ice, -oke, and -ump, which appear in over 500 words commonly used in children's early reading books. Once children have grasped the idea that words that share sounds (onsets or rimes) often share the same spelling, they can use this understanding to help them to read unknown words. This process whereby knowledge of one word guides the reading of another, similarly spelt, word is called reading by analogy. By knowing how to read the words *fish* and *dish* for example, a child may make an educated guess as to how to read the unknown word *wish*.

Children can do this from the earliest stages of reading acquisition, but the sophistication and accuracy of their analogies develops with reading experience. Inexperienced readers might only be able to draw fairly obvious analogies between words such as *peak* and *beak* that share the same rime (*eak*), but more experienced readers will also draw analogies between words such as *peak*, *peal*, and *peace* that share the same onset and the initial part of the rime (*pea*).

A study looking at the use of analogy in reading asked seven- and ten-year-old children and adults to read lists of made-up non-words. These non-words were created so that they could be read either 'phonetically' (using grapheme-phoneme correspondence rules to sound out the words) or 'by analogy' (pronouncing them in the same way as real words that share a similar spelling). The word *tepherd*, for example, could be read as 'tefferd' (phonetically) or as 'tep-herd' (by analogy with the word *shepherd*). This study found that the seven-year-old children made very little use of analogy, reading only 14% of the unknown words this way. The ten-year-old children read 34% of the unknown words by analogy with real words, a figure very close to the adult figure of 38%. These results suggest that even though the youngest children in this study were able to use analogy to support their reading of some unknown non-words, this ability develops with age and reading experience as familiarity with words increases. It is possible in this study, for example, that the seven-year-old children were unfamiliar with the written word *shepherd* so were unable to use this word to aid in their reading of *tepherd*. By the age of ten years, however, children's knowledge of words has increased considerably and their use of analogy is almost at an adult level.

Just because children are able to read unfamiliar words by analogy to familiar words does not mean that they do this spontaneously, however. Some research has shown that children are more likely to read non-words and unfamiliar real words by grapheme-phoneme conversion than they are to read by analogy unless the use of analogy is explicitly encouraged.

Learning to spell

Up to this point the focus has been on how children learn to read. But this is only part of the story. As children learn to read they also, usually, learn to spell. However, the two functions are different and it is not uncommon for people to develop into good readers but extremely poor spellers, as Joy Pollock writes:

> In the past, children have been told that the more they read the better they will be able to spell. But for many people this is just not true. A woman, 45 years old, coming for spelling lessons once said that she had been reading for forty years and was still unable to write many words correctly.
>
> *Day-to-Day Dyslexia in the Classroom* by Joy Pollock, Elisabeth Waller, and Rody Politt, p. 65

Research with young children indicates that their earliest attempts at spelling generally involve the fairly random use of upper and lower case letters, numbers, and letter-like symbols to represent words. Although this stage of development has been labelled *pre-communicative* or *pre-alphabetic*, the child is clearly able to demonstrate some rudimentary knowledge of the alphabet. However, this knowledge does not extend to their writing particular letters to represent particular sounds. So, for example, a child may write something approximating 'Ln' to represent the spoken word *cat*, while 'Py3lly' may represent *dog* (clearly, these letters and numbers in no way spell out *cat* or *dog* but at this stage the child has no knowledge of which letters represent which sounds). At this stage children may be able to read (to recognise) visually distinctive words – such as *school* – that they are unable to spell.

Once children are introduced to the names and sounds of the letters of the alphabet in a structured way, this (usually) brings about a rapid awareness that individual letters can represent individual sounds. Children's spellings subsequently begin to change to reflect this awareness, and it is not uncommon for them to be able to spell regular words that they cannot yet read. However, they have not yet fully grasped the idea that all sounds must be represented in the spelling of a word so that, for example, 'mk' may be written for 'milk' or 'dgy' for 'doggy'. Children are also prone to use letter names to represent spoken sounds, for example writing 'AT' for 'eighty', or 'U' for 'you' (an increasingly common spelling of the word 'you' by the SMS text generation). For fairly obvious reasons, this is termed the *semi-phonetic* or *partial alphabetic* stage.

By the *phonetic* or *full alphabetic* stage children are aware that all of the sounds in words need to be represented by letters in a systematic way. However, their still limited experience of spelling in a complex language such as English, where one sound may be written in many different ways, can result in them producing incorrect, although generally plausible, spellings such as 'frend' and 'telifone'.

As children progress through this stage they gradually stop producing phonetic spellings and move towards correct spelling.

Even words that are spelt incorrectly will generally tend to conform to the permissible spelling rules of the language. This is known as a *transitional* stage before children reach the final *correct* or *consolidated alphabetic* stage where their spellings are firmly rooted in the rules, or the orthography, of their language. By this time, familiar words and unfamiliar words are spelt more accurately; knowledge of prefixes (e.g. *dis-* or *un-*) and suffixes (e.g. *-able* or *-ful*) is developing; and subtle rules for spelling potentially problematic words, such as *separate* and *tomorrow*, are being learned (the word *separate*, for example, contains 'a rat', while *tomorrow* may be remembered as 'Tom'-'orrow').

The interplay between reading and spelling

Reading and spelling usually develop out of step with each other even though the two skills are clearly inter-related and mutually facilitating. At different stages of development children will be able to read words that they cannot spell and spell words that they cannot read. The development of skills in one domain, however, encourages the development of those same skills in the other domain.

As children learn the alphabet for reading they also start to write simple words. This spelling practice, in turn, increases the children's alphabetic knowledge, which increases their reading ability. Once they have mastered the fundamental skills of letter-by-letter reading, children progress to reading based on larger chunks of letters. They start reading by analogy, their orthographic skills develop, and reading becomes a gradually more automatic process. This improvement in reading ability also, usually, improves the children's spelling ability.

But not all children necessarily follow the same path from novice to skilled reader/speller. The cognitive mechanisms that underlie these various stages are not always clearly defined and it is difficult to see how any one model could adequately explain the development of reading and spelling across languages, schools, teaching methods, and individuals.

While models of reading and spelling *development* differ in their descriptions of the stages that children pass through as they learn to read and spell, there is far greater agreement about the processes underlying *skilled* reading and spelling.

Models of skilled reading and spelling

It is suggested that skilled readers read single words (in alphabetic languages) by following one of two routes:

1. By identifying them by sight as whole units – this is called the lexical route, although it is also sometimes referred to as the semantic route, or reading by eye.
2. By identifying them through grapheme-phoneme conversion – this is called the sub-lexical route, although it is also known as the phonological route, or reading by ear.

This is the *dual route* model of reading, illustrated in figure 2.

Reading via the lexical route involves recognising familiar regular and irregular printed words as whole entities from among the store of known words in the mental lexicon (this can be thought of as a mental dictionary). When you look up a word, for example the word *badger*, in a dictionary, you gain access to its phonetic pronunciation – 'BAJ-er' with the stress on the capitalised letters; you are also told what type of word it is – a 'noun'; and you are given a definition – something along the lines of 'a heavy-set, nocturnal mammal, of the *Mustelidae* family; has grey and black fur on its body with black and white stripes on its head'. Similarly, when a reader sees a familiar word

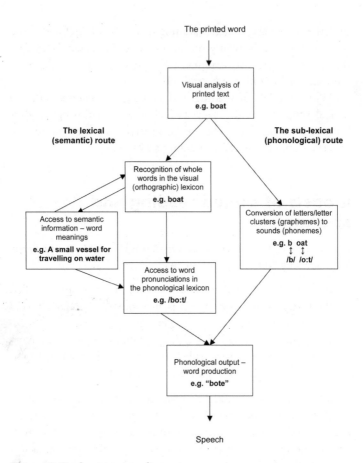

Figure 2 Dual routes to reading

that is represented in their mental lexicon they are able to access its pronunciation and meaning. Of course, unfamiliar words will not be represented within the lexicon so they will not be read via this route.

By contrast, reading via the sub-lexical route involves convert-ing printed letters and groups of letters (e.g. 'tion' or 'ing') into their corresponding sounds according to grapheme-phoneme rules. For example, to read the unfamiliar word *cat* a child must first convert the printed word into its corresponding sounds 'k', 'a', 't'. Think about the way that you would read out the word *dodecahedron* and you will, in all likelihood, use this same process. This route to reading enables us to read regular words, unfamiliar words and pronounceable non-words (e.g. *caplot*), although we would quickly come unstuck trying to read irregular words, such as *chord* or *aisle*, via this route.

The development of dual route models of reading arose largely from observation of patients with acquired dyslexia. Some patients appeared unable to recognise words as whole units. Instead, they decoded words by applying grapheme-phoneme correspondence rules. They were better able to read regular words and nonsense words (e.g. *plenk* and *trode*) than irregular real words (e.g. *pint*, which would be read as if it rhymed with *mint* and *glint*). This pattern of errors suggested that these patients were relying exclusively on the sub-lexical route to reading after the lexical route had been impaired.

By contrast, other acquired dyslexia patients could read familiar words as whole units but they were unable to read by applying grapheme-phoneme correspondence rules. They were better at reading regular and irregular familiar words (e.g. *cat* and *cough*) than unfamiliar words or orthographically acceptable nonsense words (e.g. *tonquil*). This pattern suggests that patients are relying exclusively on the lexical route to reading following impairment to the sub-lexical route.

Models of skilled spelling tend to be very similar to dual route models of reading. One route – the sub-lexical route – involves the conversion of individual sounds into their corresponding letters according to our knowledge of the phoneme-grapheme (sound-spelling) rules of our language. The other route mirrors the lexical route of reading in that the pronunciation of the word to be spelt provides access to the mental lexicon in which the individual is able to 'look up' the correct sequence of letters required to spell the word.

The ability to read does not exist in isolation from the child's many other skills and abilities. Different skills appear to be of critical importance at different stages of reading and spelling development, and for skilled reading. Individual differences in these skills may account for variations in the *rate* and *success* of a child's reading development. As you may well have realised from reading the descriptions of the models above, awareness of the sounds of the spoken language, and of how these are represented by letters in the written language, are of primary importance for reading and spelling. This is encapsulated by the term *phonological awareness*. Children develop phonological awareness through experience of spoken language and through explicit phonics-based reading instruction.

Phonological awareness and phonics

Phonological awareness is the conscious ability to recognise (and manipulate) individual sounds in spoken language, from words to syllables, rhymes, onsets, rimes, and phonemes. This awareness develops along a continuum which Professor Marilyn Jager Adams identified as consisting of five levels. From the simplest to the most difficult, these levels of phonological awareness are:

• Awareness of rhyme and alliteration.
  The simplest forms of phonological awareness involve hearing individual words within sentences, and identifying alliteration and rhyme. These skills, which provide the foundation for the child's reading ability, usually develop in the pre-school years through learning nursery rhymes and playing games involving naming words that start with the same sound.

- Explicit awareness of shared sounds within words.
  Once children have mastered the fundamental skills of rhyme and alliteration, they are then able to distinguish between words that share the same sounds and those that don't. The shared sound may be at the start of the word (e.g. the words *sun*, *sock*, and *sad* share the same first sound which the word *box* does not), or at the end of the word (e.g. the words *bat*, *cat*, and *mat* share the same last sound which the word *fan* does not).
- The ability to divide and blend syllables.
  The next level of phonological awareness sees the child dividing words into syllables (e.g. *donkey* to 'don' and 'key'), onsets and rimes (e.g. 'd' and 'onkey'), and blending syllables to produce words (e.g. joining together 'win' and 'dow' to produce 'window').
- The ability to segment phonemes.
  By this stage of development children are able to divide words and syllables into their individual sounds (phonemes), such that the word *donkey* may be segmented into the phonemes 'd', 'o', 'n', 'k', 'ee'. Children at this stage are able to count and identify the phonemes within words.
- The ability to manipulate phonemes.
  Once children have learned that spoken words and syllables can be sub-divided in different ways, they can use this understanding to manipulate words by adding sounds (adding 't' to *able* to form *table*), deleting sounds (removing 'k' from *milk* to produce *mill*), or swapping sounds (swapping the initial sounds of the words *pink* and *men* to form 'mink' and 'pen').

Phonics

The importance of phonology is highlighted in a method of teaching called phonics which is designed to make explicit the link between letters/letter strings and the sounds that they represent. There are two types of phonics teaching methods: synthetic phonics and analytic phonics.

Synthetic phonics involves teaching children the forty-four sounds that make up all the words of spoken English. Letter sounds are taught rather than letter names, so a 'd' would be taught as a 'duh' not a 'dee'. Children are then shown how to blend these sounds together to form complete words. Five or six letter sounds are taught per week and children are encouraged to produce and pronounce words for themselves based on their letter sound knowledge.

One of the most widely used commercial phonics schemes is called *Jolly Phonics* (other phonics schemes/resources have the wonderfully alliterative names *Fast Phonics First*, *FastTrack Phonics* and *Fishy Phonics*). In the Jolly Phonics scheme the sounds of the language are taught in groups of seven that can easily be blended together to make simple words. The sounds are written either as individual letters (e.g. 's', 'a', 't') or letter pairs (e.g. 'oa', 'ie', 'ng'), and they are taught in a multi-sensory way associating each sound with an action, for example making an 'S' shape with the hands, like a snake, while making a 'ssss' sound.

Analytic phonics is a different approach in that reading is initially taught by presenting children with whole words to help them to build up a sight vocabulary. Letter names (in preference to letter sounds) are then taught gradually over a period of two years. Children are encouraged to focus on initial letters to help them to guess at the identities of unfamiliar words. Once children have developed this early sight vocabulary, they may be shown clusters of whole words and taught how to break them down into their component parts, such as the onset and rime. These words might share common initial letters (e.g. *milk*, *make*, and *man*) or common rimes (e.g. *park*, *lark*, and *mark*). Children are introduced to words in books and encouraged to attempt to read unfamiliar words based on the context and pictures in the book.

A 2006 review of the teaching of early reading (called *the Rose report*) assessed the efficacy of phonics-based reading schemes. This review found that the teaching of phonics is an essential part of reading instruction, noting that:

> the teaching of phonic work must teach beginner readers to process all the letters in words and 'read words in and out of text'. Because our writing system is alphabetic, beginner readers will not become skilled and fluent, comprehending readers and writers if they cannot understand and operate the system. The case for systematic phonic work is therefore overwhelming.

Furthermore, on the basis of evidence regarding the relative merits of synthetic and analytic phonics schemes – gathered from teachers, researchers, school inspectors, and government departments responsible for standards in education – the review found that:

> there is much convincing evidence to show ... that, as generally understood, 'synthetic' phonics is the form of systematic phonic work that offers the vast majority of beginners the best route to becoming skilled readers.

The review recommended, therefore, the use of synthetic phonics as the more effective first-line teaching approach for all children by the age of five.

Phonics and the teaching of reading

In a report published in 2000, the US National Reading Panel – a group of literacy experts – assessed the effectiveness of various methods of reading instruction. They identified phonological awareness and phonics, alongside fluency, vocabulary, and text comprehension, as crucial skills for reading proficiency.

The No Child Left Behind Act (2001; successor to the Elementary and Secondary Education Act, 1965) places similar emphasis on the teaching of language and literacy skills, and requires that all children be reading at an age-appropriate level (or above) by the school year 2013–14. Although the mechanics of the instructional programme are not specified at a national level (there is no national curriculum for reading), the Act states that all children should have access to 'effective, scientifically based instructional strategies' (Section 1001 [9]). These strategies take the form of the Early Reading First programme for pre-school-age children, and the Reading First programme for elementary school-age children (US Department of Education, 2001). Instruction in these programmes has the teaching of phonemic awareness and phonics at its core. Schools are required to meet State goals for achievement (to demonstrate 'adequate yearly progress'), particularly for students from low income families, for those from racial and ethnic sub-groups, and for those with disabilities. Federal funding depends on reaching these targets.

Reading achievement is tested each year in the United States as part of the National Assessment of Educational Progress (NAEP). The results of this assessment are reported in a document colloquially referred to as 'the nation's report card'. At each grade level, a child's reading ability is classified as:

1. Basic, if he/she demonstrates a literal understanding of the meaning of age-appropriate text.
2. Proficient, if he/she is also able to infer meaning from text.
3. Advanced, if he/she demonstrates superior reading and comprehension skills, including an ability to evaluate text critically, and to generalise about topics presented in the text.

Results reported in 2007 showed the following results for

nine-year-old children since the introduction of the No Child Left behind Act in 2001:

- 8% more had reached a 'basic' level of reading; this had increased from 59% to 67%.
- 4% more had reached a 'proficient' level of reading; this had increased from 29% to 33%.
- 1% more had reached an 'advanced' level of reading; this had increased from 7% to 8%.

However, the results for thirteen year olds over this same period were less encouraging. Of these children:

- 1% more had reached a 'basic' level of reading; this had increased from 73% to 74%.
- 1% fewer had reached a 'proficient' level of reading; this had decreased from 32% to 31%.
- There was no change in the numbers who had reached an 'advanced' level of reading; this figure stayed at a constant 3%.

In England the National Literacy Strategy (Department for Education and Employment, 1998) and its successor, the Primary Framework for Literacy and Mathematics (2006) requires that all primary schools spend an hour each day ('the literacy hour') teaching a structured programme of reading-related skills. The Primary Framework for Literacy and Mathematics built upon this strategy by emphasising the importance of effective, systematic phonics-based instruction in the teaching of reading, writing, speaking, and listening. Strict targets were set within each of these strategies for primary schools to raise the standards of literacy of their pupils, and these seem to be having some effect. In 1998 only 65% of eleven-year-old children were reading at an age-appropriate level. By 2005 this figure was nearly 80% for the eleven-year-old children whose schooling had started with the introduction of the National Literacy Strategy in 1998.

As we have seen, children need to achieve a certain level of phonological awareness if they are to learn to read and spell normally. Some phonological awareness will come from their pre-school experience of reciting nursery rhymes and singing rhyming songs; other phonological awareness will only develop after the child has learned that the sounds of spoken words may be represented in a systematic way by individual letters or groups of letters.

Testing time after time ...

One way of exploring the relationship between phonological awareness and reading is to test children's phonological aware-ness before they learn to read, and then to test reading ability several months, or even years, later. If children with good phonological awareness at the first time of testing become good readers at the second time of testing, while children with initially poor phonological awareness go on to become poor readers, then it seems reasonable to assume that early phonological awareness is important for later reading development.

Studies have shown that simple phonological awareness measured in pre-literate kindergarten children is a good predic-tor of later reading ability. Children with good awareness in kindergarten develop into good readers while those with poor awareness struggle to become skilled readers. Tests of phono-logical awareness that predict reading typically require the reader to produce rhymes (e.g. what words rhyme with *pin*?) or to blend individual spoken sound into a single word (e.g. what word do you get if you add 'm' onto *ice*?). But why should pre-literate children's ability to produce rhymes or to blend sounds predict their later reading development?

The simple skills that children learn from playing with sounds in this way represent their first steps towards developing phonological awareness. Children are encouraged by their parents and teachers to recite nursery rhymes, sing alphabetic songs, and play games with sounds (e.g. a snake makes a 'sssss' sound; what sound does a bee make?). As this progresses, they become increasingly aware of the individual sounds within the spoken language. Their attention will be drawn to similarities and differences in these sounds and to ways in which these sounds can be manipulated. The skills that children acquire through these simple activities underpin the development of increasingly sophisticated phonological awareness that will form the building blocks of reading and spelling development. However, this is only part of a rather more complex story.

A child's phonological awareness consistently predicts his/her future reading ability but reading ability also predicts a child's future phonological awareness. As their reading skills develop, children become increasingly aware of the letter sequences in words. This feeds back into their phonological awareness by enabling them to develop more sophisticated phonological skills. For example, the ability to delete individual sounds from words (e.g. what word do you get if you take away the 'l' sound from *leg*?) and to substitute phonemes within words (e.g. what word do you get if you replace the 'f' of *fish* with a 'd'?). In this way, early phonological awareness supports the learning of early reading skills, while experience with reading supports the further development of phonological awareness, and so on.

From phonological awareness to reading, and back to phonological awareness

Further evidence of the importance of phonological awareness for reading development comes from research in which children are taught phonological awareness skills over a period of time while the effect of this training on their subsequent reading ability is monitored. Other children receive no phonological awareness training during this period. If the reading ability of the children who receive training increases to a greater degree than that of the children who receive no training, then it may be concluded that the phonological skills that are taught influence later reading development.

In one of the earliest and most extensive studies of this kind, groups of non-reading (pre-literate) children with poor phonological awareness were trained over two years either in rhyme and alliteration or in the categorisation of objects (e.g. a hen might be categorised either as an animal or as a farm animal). Children in the 'categorisation' group received no phonological training. Tests of reading and spelling ability at the end of the training period revealed that children who had received phonological awareness training were better (more accurate) readers and spellers than were those who had received no phonological training.

At a more naturalistic level, a pre-literate child's knowledge of nursery rhymes is an extremely accurate predictor of their rhyme awareness and reading ability at the end of their first year of school. This effect is thought to occur in two ways:

1. Young children who can detect the rhyming words in nursery rhymes are already able to hear the onsets and rimes within these words,

   e.g. 'Humpty Dumpty sat on a wall' (onset = 'w'; rime = 'all')

   'Humpty Dumpty had a great fall' (onset = 'f'; rime = 'all')

   These children go on to learn how to sub-divide the onset and rime into their individual sounds (phonemes), and awareness of phonemes underpins success in reading and spelling.

2. Novice readers quickly become aware that many words that rhyme (e.g. *make, take, lake*) are spelt in a consistent way.

This awareness enables them, implicitly, to categorise written words with shared sounds. Making this awareness explicit through reading and spelling instruction – for example, teaching that words that end with an 'ake' sound share the written letter sequence 'ake' – boosts children's reading and spelling development as they learn to read and spell unfamiliar words by analogy with similarly spelt familiar words.

Some aspects of phonological awareness develop before reading instruction while others emerge as children's reading skills develop. Research into the effects of different types of reading instruction on children's later phonological awareness has shown that children who receive phonics-based instruction are better at identifying and manipulating sounds within words than are children whose reading instruction involves learning to recognise whole words (the so-called 'look-say' approach).

As we have seen throughout this chapter, there are many different aspects of phonological awareness, such as awareness of rhyme and alliteration, the ability to divide and blend syllables, and the ability to segment phonemes. So, considering phonological awareness as a single entity, and as either a prerequisite to reading, or a result of reading, is far too simplistic. Instead it may be that some degree of ability to reflect on spoken words, possibly at the level of the onset and rime, is necessary – but not necessarily *sufficient* – to gain a fundamental appreciation of the spelling rules of alphabetic languages. The ability to break words down into onsets and rimes aids basic word recognition and represents the first step in the foundation of a sight vocabulary. As this sight vocabulary expands, the child focuses increasingly on the sounds of words and becomes gradually more aware that onsets and rimes may be decomposed into smaller units (individual phonemes). The increasing complexity of a child's reflections on spoken words feeds into his/her reading skills which in turn bring about more complex forms of phonological awareness.

In this chapter we've seen how reading develops by following an expected path alongside the development of phonological awareness, with children becoming gradually aware of smaller and smaller sounds within spoken and written words – from the whole word to syllables, onsets and rimes, and individual phonemes/graphemes. A pre-reading child's phonological awareness provides a clear prediction of their later reading and spelling ability such that children with good phonological awareness develop into good readers. Of course, some children have extremely poor phonological awareness and develop into extremely poor readers. The role of phonological awareness in dyslexia is explored in the next chapter.

3

The importance of sound in reading

Having made a strenuous effort to understand the symbols he could make nothing of, he [Gustave Flaubert] wept giant tears … For a long time he could not understand the elementary connection that made of two letters one-syllable, of several syllables a word

Caroline Commanville (Flaubert's niece)

Dyslexia has been likened to an iceberg. The tip of the iceberg – the overt reading difficulty – is visible, but more problems lie unseen below the surface. Since the 1990s there have been considerable advances in uncovering the body of this iceberg. One of the most important advances has been the identification of problems people have in analysing and manipulating the sound of words. When children with these problems start school and begin reading and spelling instruction in alphabetic languages, they experience difficulty with:

1. perceiving the sounds of individual letters and syllables within spoken words (phonological processing);
2. recognising when words, such as *chair* and *bear*, rhyme (rhyme awareness);
3. providing words that rhyme with other words; for example, words that rhyme with *park* (rhyme production);
4. counting the number of different sounds within words, such as the three sounds – 'r', 'ay', 's' – in the word 'race' (phoneme segmentation);

5. deciding if words, such as *fish* and *phone*, start with the same sound (alliterative awareness);
6. learning the relationship between written letters and the sounds that they represent (learning letter-sound, or grapheme-phoneme, correspondences);
7. naming objects, numbers, and colours quickly (rapid automatic naming);
8. repeating spoken words such as *honorarium*, and non-words such as *trembut* (verbal repetition);
9. remembering lists of words – such as days of the week or months of the year – in the correct order (verbal sequencing);
10. developing a spoken vocabulary.

These difficulties underlie the *phonological deficit* theory of dyslexia.

The effect of phonological deficits on someone's ability to read will depend to a great extent on the language that they speak. In alphabetic languages such as English, individual spoken sounds are represented by individual letters or groups of letters. To learn to read and spell a young child must learn the complex rules by which these letters and sounds relate to each other. In non-alphabetic, logographic languages such as Chinese, written characters represent whole syllables or even whole words. There is no need to break words down into individual phonemes either in reading or spelling. Phonological impairments have the potential to cause greater difficulty (and lead to a higher incidence of dyslexia) in alphabetic languages than in logographic languages.

However, the story is not quite that simple. As you saw in chapter 1, some alphabetic languages such as English and Danish are complex and irregular while others, such as Italian and Serbo-Croatian, are highly regular. Children learning to read regular languages, even those with poor phonological skills, experience relatively little difficulty with learning the spelling-sound rules of the language; the prevalence of developmental dyslexia in these languages is relatively low. Conversely, children learning to read irregular languages experience great difficulty with learning the spelling-sound rules of the language if their phonological skills are impaired; the prevalence of developmental dyslexia in these languages is relatively high. (This topic is considered in more detail in chapter 5.)

Deficiency or delay?

Explanations for the source of dyslexic readers' phonological impairments have focused primarily on notions of:

1. Deficiency – These phonological problems are the result of fundamental *deficiencies*, so dyslexic readers will never achieve good phonological awareness no matter how hard they try.
2. Delay – These phonological problems are the result of developmental *delays*, so dyslexic readers may take longer than non-dyslexic readers to develop phonological awareness but eventually they will develop good phonological skills.

Support for the deficiency hypothesis comes from observations that whereas the phonological skills of non-dyslexic readers improve with age and reading experience, dyslexic readers don't show this same improvement. They perform more poorly on tasks of phonological awareness than do non-dyslexic readers of the same age, and more poorly than non-dyslexic readers of the same reading age. (An eight-year-old dyslexic reader may have a reading age of six years.)

One study of early language development in children with at least one dyslexic parent tested language skills in these children from the age of two-and-a-half to eight years. At the age of eight, 65% of these children with a family history of dyslexia were identified as dyslexic, compared with 5% of children with no family history of dyslexia. Retrospective examination of the language abilities of the two groups revealed that those children who 'became' dyslexic were distinguishable from children who developed into unimpaired readers in the following ways:

- At the age of two-and-a-half years they produced shorter, less complex sentences; they also mispronounced more words in their spontaneous speech.
- At three years they displayed a poorer vocabulary – they understood the meanings of fewer words, and they were less able to provide the names of objects.
- At five years they were less able to name written letters, to provide the sounds that these letters represent, to name objects, and they displayed poorer phonological awareness.

This suggests that the language difficulties associated with dyslexia are present from a very young age. Studies with older children and adults show that dyslexic readers' difficulties in recognising words, in spelling, and in phonological processing persist throughout childhood and into adulthood, even in individuals whose reading ability has developed, through training, to an age-appropriate level.

While dyslexic readers eventually learn to recognise some words by sight, this may be predominantly through the use of a look and say approach – with repeated exposure to common words, children learn to recognise their shape as a whole. Take this example from a dyslexic boy called Paul:

> I remember words by the pattern of the letters. With a word like 'sugar' I remember that it has a flat-topped shape so I know that it hasn't got a tall letter in it and it can't be 'sh' at the beginning although it sounds as though it should be. I see the outline shapes of words so when I look at a page I see the words as patterns. When I do manage to really learn a word, I throw the shape away and just keep the word in my mind.

> *The Reality of Dyslexia* by John Osmond, p. 27

So, in the absence of efficient grapheme-phoneme conversion skills, dyslexic readers are still able to read some common words – such as 'the', 'on', 'a', 'was' – accurately by sight. They read less familiar words, however, by guessing, guided by the word's context. These guesses are often incorrect and the spoken words bear little resemblance to the written words. For example, the following is the original text shown to a dyslexic girl called Sarah:

> Now the children were discussing their new play. 'We need a brave person for the mountain rescue', explained a boy. Each puppet tried to appear like the required hero. Then cheers greeted the boy's choice. On the stage was raised the shy but happy Swiss puppet.

But this is how Sarah read the text:

> How the children were designing their new play. 'We need a brave man of the mount chishime', ixslating a boy. Each puppy tried to apprat the real heeyou. The chance great the boy's chorus. On to the stage was realized the scene but happy Swizz puppy.

> *Overcoming Dyslexia* by Bevé Hornsby, p. 28

Reading for non-dyslexic children is likely to be enjoyable, and so they will happily spend time doing it. This has the effect of boosting children's reading fluency, their vocabulary, and comprehension. This phenomenon, where reading success leads to further reading success, is called *cumulative achievement*.

Dyslexic children, however, tend to follow a rather different path. For these children poor phonological awareness hampers their understanding of the rules of reading and writing and, in general, their reading is a slow, inaccurate, and laborious process. This is clearly demonstrated by the following recollection of a dyslexic woman, identified only as 'X', that was printed in a scientific journal in 1936:

> My mother offered to give me ten shillings if I would read a book. I tried to get through 'Black Beauty'. I was devoted to horses and this book about a pony attracted me. I worked away at it alone and with the governess month after month. I made a little 'V' on the page to show how far I had got – I never finished the book or, of course, received the ten shillings, and 'Black Beauty' is a nightmare to me.
>
> *British Journal of Ophthalmology*, 20, 2, p. 74

Although the particular abilities of dyslexic children vary, for most reading is often less than enjoyable and they avoid it wherever possible. This is summed up in the following description of one dyslexic boy's feelings towards reading:

> Bradley often hears his mum say, 'It's a great day to curl up on the sofa with a good book', but reading has always been more pain than pleasure for Bradley. Curling up with a book has never been a positive experience for him ... For Bradley, reading is the worst form of punishment; he'd rather clean both his room and his rabbit's cage than curl up on the sofa with a good book.
>
> *The Secret Life of the Dyslexic Child* by Robert Frank, p. 50

Poor readers in primary school, like Bradley, read on average around 100,000 words per year, significantly fewer than the ten million words read by good readers. This relative lack of reading experience hampers the development of their vocabulary, their reading fluency, comprehension, and general knowledge. This phenomenon, called *cumulative impoverishment*, has been named the Matthew effect, from the Parable of the Talents related in the Gospel according to St Matthew (25:29):

> For everyone who has will be given more, and he will have an abundance. Whoever does not have, even what he has will be taken from him.

Difficulty with auditory discrimination

It is possible, of course, that the phonological difficulties of dyslexia are just part of a broader problem with the processing of sounds. Research has shown that many dyslexic readers are poorer than non-dyslexic readers at distinguishing between pairs of simple tones (beeps) that are presented in quick succession. The dyslexic readers require a longer gap to be left between the presentation of the two tones − hundreds of milliseconds − before they are able to hear that there are two tones instead of just one. Non-dyslexic readers require a gap of tens of milliseconds, i.e. one tenth the gap required by dyslexic readers.

A similar phenomenon is found for rapidly presented speech sounds, such as 'ba' and 'da'. Dyslexic readers need a much longer gap between the two speech sounds before they are able to hear them as being distinct. This has clear implications for dyslexic readers' ability to process spoken language. If they have difficulty differentiating between the spoken words *bat, cat,* and *mat,* this will hinder the development of their phonological processing ability and will cause problems with their reading development.

A study by Elise Temple and colleagues at Stanford University set out to test this hypothesis. Dyslexic children were provided with intensive training in auditory discrimination for 100 minutes a day, five days a week for eight weeks. During this time, children completed exercises (presented as computer games) which involved:

- distinguishing between similar speech sounds;
- identifying the odd-word-out from sequences of words that differed in their first or final sounds;
- matching speech sounds;
- matching words to pictures of the objects that they represent

(e.g. children were shown a picture of a boy and a toy and asked to point to the toy).

In these tasks the speech was artificially slowed down and amplified so that children were able to hear clearly the differences between similar-sounding words. As the training progressed, the speed of the voice was increased gradually.

At the end of the training period the dyslexic children's reading of real words and non-words had improved significantly, as had their comprehension and their ability to name digits, letters, objects, and colours rapidly. The authors point out, however, that while the group as a whole showed improvements, the result hides a large amount of variability – some children showed dramatic improvement post-training, others showed no improvement at all.

This issue of variability within groups of dyslexic readers is important as other research shows that not all dyslexic readers have difficulty distinguishing between rapidly presented sounds, either speech sounds or non-speech sounds. In fact, only around 50% do. This figure indicates that problems with the rapid processing of speech sounds do not cause reading difficulties for many dyslexic children. Whether they cause reading difficulties in a sub-set of these children is unknown.

Verbal memory problems

A good memory helps a child to link the sounds of spoken language with their written forms. It also underpins the learning of vocabulary and the development of general language skills such as comprehension. It is easy to see how problems with memory might seriously hamper a child's reading development.

Imagine that you are a young child who has been receiving reading lessons in school. You have been learning the sounds

Symbol	Sound	Symbol	Sound	Symbol	Sound
~	/b/ as in bag	#	/m/ as in mouse	-	/x/ as in box
!	/c/ as in cat	±	/n/ as in nose	≠	/y/ as in yell
%	/d/ as in dog	+	/p/ as in pig	π	/z/ as in zoo
)	/f/ as in fish	=	/q/ as in queen		
^	/g/ as in glue	?	/r/ as in run	}	/a/ as in bat
$	/h/ as in hat	¢	/s/ as in star	√	/e/ as in led
@	/j/ as in jump	∝	/t/ as in tap	≈	/i/ as in fit
&	/k/ as in kitten	÷	/v/ as in voice	¿	/o/ as in pot
*	/l/ as in lemon	«	/w/ as in wall	§	/u/ as in bubble

Figure 3a An artificial reading task

that are associated with printed symbols. These printed symbols, and the sounds they represent, are shown in figure 3a.

After a few lessons you are asked to read out the short passage of simple text in figure 3b. Use the key (figure 3a) if this helps.

∝$√ ~*}!& !}∝

@}±√ ¢}≈%, "*¿¿& }∝ ∝$≈¢ *≈∝∝*√ ~*}!& !}∝."

"¿$", ¢}≈% ¢}?}$, "≈∝ ≈¢ ¢¿ ¢#}**.

«√ #§¢∝ ∝}&√ ≈∝ $¿#√ ∝¿ #¿∝$√?"

Figure 3b An artificial reading task

This is a tedious task and should give you some idea of the difficulty (and resulting panic) faced by dyslexic readers. Not only do you have to recognise the individual symbols and convert these into their corresponding sounds, you then need to remember these sounds and blend them together into complete words, while trying to remember individual words in order to make sense of the text.

You might have realised from this little exercise that even having the 'key' in front of you doesn't always help that much. The way the individual letters are pronounced in the story is not always the same as the pronunciations you have learned from the keywords. In fact, not many of these words are strictly decodable on the basis of the letter-sound rules that you have been taught (the word 'it' being one of the few exceptions). This irregularity of the English language is a recurring theme throughout this book, and it is a constant source of difficulty for dyslexic readers. And in case you are still wondering, the English 'translation' of this passage is shown in figure 3c.

The black cat

Jane said, "Look at this little black cat."

"Oh", said Sarah, "it is so small.

We must take it home to mother"

Figure 3c An artificial reading task

Memory difficulties have been linked to developmental dyslexia. Dyslexic children and adults often have problems, for example, remembering:

- telephone numbers;
- multiplication tables;
- directions – which is left and which is right;
- days of the week;
- arithmetic symbols, particularly remembering the difference between similar-looking ones, such as + and x, or − and ÷;
- people's names;
- dates and times of appointments;
- nursery rhymes or poems;
- dialogue for a play;
- dates of birth (even their own).

The daily difficulties caused by these memory problems are reflected in this passage by a dyslexic boy called Steven:

> I have a lack of short-term memory. I just can't remember random sets of numbers. I was sixteen before I knew all the months of the year in order ... I go cold every time I see a form ... I can't remember an address if someone gives it to me or a telephone number ... If I'm in the middle of taking notes and something else intervenes ... then I easily get lost. Remembering the next sentence when you've looked down from the board is almost impossible when you are three or four sentences behind trying to keep up and trying to listen to someone at the same time.

> *The Reality of Dyslexia* by John Osmond, p. 32

And in the following way by a dyslexic woman called Peggy:

> If I've got two or three calls to make in town, I've got to write down the places I'm going to, or I shall go right by them. Um, you know, I mean people can usually remember that they're going to go to the post office, then they've got to call at the butcher's, then they're going to go to the library. I can set off and I'll miss the library, or miss the post office. I just walk right

by because I don't remember … step-by-step things that I'm doing.

Dyslexia, the Self and Higher Education by David Pollak, p. 171

Learning vocabulary is also difficult for dyslexic readers, a problem described by five times Olympic gold medallist rower, Sir Steve Redgrave:

> When I was a child, dyslexia was only starting to be used as a name – we didn't really know what it was. I was taken out of doing French and English lessons – if you're struggling with your own language what is the point in doing another?

Similarly, Charles Schwab, billionaire businessman and philanthropist, recalls his struggle with language at Stanford University:

> I flunked English twice. They just passed me through the third time. I got an F in French. I had a tough enough time with the first language.

Dyslexic readers' memory difficulties are not restricted to printed text but they do tend to have more difficulty remembering verbal than pictorial material. In one study of verbal memory, dyslexic and non-dyslexic university students were asked to listen to and repeat four sentences of increasing length and complexity (from 'Billy has made a beautiful boat out of wood with his sharp knife' to 'At the end of the week the newspaper published a complete account of the experiences of the great explorer'). If the student repeated the sentence correctly, he/she moved on to the next sentence. If it was repeated incorrectly, he/she listened to the same sentence again and was asked to repeat it. Whereas the non-dyslexic readers required the sentences to be repeated a total of 125 times (no one individual required more than eight repetitions), the dyslexic readers required 902 repetitions (only six of these readers required fewer than eight repetitions). The authors suggest that this phonological weakness (difficulty remembering the precise words used, in the correct order) underlies the verbal memory problems of dyslexia.

This difficulty with remembering things in the correct order (called sequencing) is a problem for dyslexic readers. As mentioned earlier, dyslexic children commonly have problems learning the letters of the alphabet, days of the week, and months of the year in the correct order. Dyslexic readers may also have difficulty remembering sequences of verbal instructions, particularly if the instructions contain multiple steps, such as 'Go and fetch your gloves and scarf from the cupboard upstairs, then come back down and put your coat and shoes on'. Many parents and teachers of dyslexic children will be familiar with the experience of asking the children to do something, only to be asked again a few minutes later 'What was it you wanted me to do?'

While dyslexic readers commonly have poor memory for verbal material, their memory for non-verbal material, such as unfamiliar faces, abstract designs, or visual patterns, is generally no worse than that of non-dyslexic readers. As you will see in the next chapter, it may even be better.

Different memory stores

Memory is not a single entity, and as you have just seen, people with dyslexia do not have general memory difficulties. The definition of dyslexia provided by the British Dyslexia Association specifically pointed to difficulties that dyslexic readers face with 'working memory'. This is a particular type of memory in which information is stored in the short term but we are still able to think about the information and manipulate it if necessary. For example, if you go on holiday but then want to call home, you would need to think of your telephone number, mentally delete the initial zero from the dialling code and add the international code for your country. You might then repeat this number in your head while you dial.

This operation involves working memory which is thought to comprise three components:

- the central executive, which 'oversees' the storage and retrieval of information;
- the visuospatial scratchpad, which is responsible for the storage of visual information. When we recall from memory a route on a map so that we can find our way to a friend's new home, this visual information is thought to be stored in the visuospatial scratchpad;
- the phonological loop, which is responsible for the storage of verbal information. When we sub-vocally rehearse an unfamiliar telephone number while we dial the phone, this verbal information is believed to be stored in the phonological loop. The operation of the phonological loop has been likened to that of a tape recorder. Verbal information is stored as a sequence of sounds, and the capacity of the loop is limited by the number of times that these sounds can be repeated in two seconds. Lists of short words (e.g. *cat*, *sit*, *hen*) are stored more easily than are lists of long words (e.g. *microphone*, *television*, *elephant*), and lists of dissimilar-sounding words (e.g. *door*, *grass*, *frog*) are stored more easily than are lists of similar-sounding words (e.g. *mat*, *pat*, *cap*).

Given the importance of phonology for the storage of verbal information in working memory, it is likely that dyslexic readers' memory difficulties are linked to their problems with phonological processing. This suggestion is supported by the finding that dyslexic readers experience particular difficulty, relative to good readers, at remembering lists of similar-sounding words such as *pin*, *bin*, *win*, *din*. Dyslexic readers' attempts at repeating lists of similar sounds under their breath, to keep the words stored in the phonological loop, tax their poor phono-logical skills too much. This in turn reduces the efficiency of their verbal memory.

A second possible explanation for the verbal memory differ-ences between good and poor readers concerns the efficiency of the individuals' memory processes. As typically developing children grow older, the amount of 'mental effort' they exert to remember and recall information decreases. These processes become more efficient with experience, so the amount of infor-mation that children are able to remember increases as they grow older. Once again, however, the poor phonological skills of dyslexic readers may reduce the efficiency of these processes, thus limiting the amount of verbal information stored in memory.

The short-term recall of information suffers as the demands of a memory task increase. For example, a simple memory task might involve asking people to remember a list of numbers, such as 6, 8, 3, 9, 1, and then repeat the numbers in the order in which they were heard (6, 8, 3, 9, 1). In a more demanding version of this task, people might be asked to recall the numbers in the correct numerical order (in this case, 1, 3, 6, 8, 9). Increasing the difficulty of the memory task in this way has a much more detrimental effect on dyslexic readers' than unimpaired readers' recall.

Similar difficulty can be experienced by a dyslexic child attempting to read an unfamiliar word, such as *follow*. To do this, they must break the word down into its constituent parts ('f', 'o', 'll', 'ow') and convert each written letter/string of letters into its corresponding sound. The child must keep the earlier sounds (e.g. 'f', 'o') in memory, as they continue to convert the rest of the word ('ll', 'ow'), before joining, or blending, these sounds together to produce a familiar word. This is a difficult task for any novice reader to perform. It is even more difficult for a novice reader with poor phonological processing skills and poor memory. While unimpaired readers eventually develop efficient, almost effortless, reading with practice, dyslexic readers continue to read slowly, with some effort, and they often have difficulty remembering what they have just read. Charles Schwab again:

> When I look at the words 'the cat crossed the street', I have to sound it out to get meaning. Most people get meaning in an automated way. Now that I'm older and focused on investments and economics, I can see some words and concepts clearly. I don't have to go through the slow manipulation in my mind. But if you gave me a book on some subject that I'm not familiar with, it would take me twice as long to read it as anybody else. Even then, I'd have a tough time answering questions on what I've read.

Another effect of poor phonological processing skills is that dyslexic readers are much slower and less accurate than non-dyslexic readers at enunciating multi-syllabic words (such as *hippopotamus*) and non-words (such as *mibrostrope*). The speed at which children are able to repeat words silently to themselves – known as rate of articulation – affects the amount of information that they are able to remember. The faster the articulation, the more frequently the word may be rehearsed, so the longer it remains in memory. Research has shown a strong relationship between reading ability, phonological processing ability, and rate of articulation; it may be that the acquisition of reading skills serves to improve articulation which in turn increases memory span.

Although dyslexic readers' memory difficulties undoubtedly contribute to their reading problems, we must not take this to mean that a poor memory causes dyslexia. While dyslexic readers are *generally* poorer on verbal memory tasks than are non-dyslexic readers, this is not always the case. Dyslexic readers' memory for non-verbal information, such as patterns, faces, or tunes, is generally found to be no different to that of non-dyslexic readers as the next chapter demonstrates.

A last word on phonology and dyslexia

When he appeared on the popular BBC Radio 4 show, *Desert Island Discs*, the writer A.A. Gill spoke of the reading problems he encountered as a result of his dyslexia. He said:

> words on a page are dried speech. They are desiccated speech
> ... you should be able to add your own head, and what you get
> back is a voice.

While this process is relatively straightforward and automatic for most people, for others it presents a daily challenge. Without knowing the recipe (the grapheme-phoneme conversion rules) by which to rehydrate this dried speech, the dyslexic reader is liable to be left to struggle without a voice.

4

Visual skill and reading ability

> Paul was almost ten years old when I found him crying over a
> spelling list. He explained that words seemed to move around
> when he tried to read, that he couldn't copy anything because
> he was unable to retain the order of the letters in his mind, and
> that he was being told to look up spellings in the dictionary but
> found it all impossible.
>
> *The Reality of Dyslexia* by John Osmond, p. 26

Historically, dyslexia was thought to be a problem caused by
difficulty in processing visual information. Morgan wrote of
'congenital word blindness' while Orton used the label
'strephosymbolia' (from the Greek words for 'turned symbols').
Both believed that dyslexic readers' difficulties primarily
manifested themselves as letter and word reversals, such that a *b*
would be read as a 'd', and *saw* would be read as 'was'. Even
today, anecdotal reports abound of letter confusions and letter
reversals in some dyslexic readers. A thirty-seven-year-old man
called Colin remembers the moment that he discovered that he
might be dyslexic:

> The man interviewing me was studying intently the paper I had
> written. Then he looked up and said … 'Have you ever consid-
> ered that you might be dyslexic?'… The man guessed I was
> dyslexic because he has a dyslexic son and my writing looked
> similar, getting my bs and ds mixed up … In one of my exami-
> nation papers I had written 'dad' for 'bad'. So I had put down

something like, 'I feel it would be dad to pursue this course at this time'.

The Reality of Dyslexia by John Osmond, p. 51

In the following example, twenty-seven-year-old Harry recalls a similar experience:

there was a little sign on the wall saying 'if you can read this, maybe you should consider, or think about dyslexia' or something. And I read it, and I thought 'well, I can read it'. I read it loads of times, and I thought 'well what's wrong with it?' And I realised 'you' was spelt the other way round; it was 'YUO'. And there was another little spelling mistake. And er it wasn't till I'd read it four or five times, I thought 'oh there's spelling mistakes in it, just switched round'. That's it. I get the message.

Dyslexia, the Self and Higher Education by David Pollak, p. 183

While children with good visual-perceptual skills experience few problems in learning to identify letter shapes, children with poorer visual skills will have problems with the perception of letters and are likely to face difficulties in learning to read. Unfortunately, although confusions due to letter reversals provide an intuitively appealing explanation for the problems experienced by dyslexic readers, evidence shows that reversal errors are actually just as likely to occur in inexperienced, non-dyslexic readers. Nevertheless, the belief that dyslexia is associated with visual-perceptual problems persists. Numerous researchers have shown that dyslexic readers perform poorly on tests of visuospatial ability, but as you will see later in the chapter, other researchers link dyslexia with visuospatial talent.

Reading weakness, visual weakness?

Dyslexic readers are often found to be poorer than non-dyslexic readers at reproducing (drawing) complex visual figures from memory, at mentally rotating letters and objects, and identifying missing elements from pictures (e.g. a picture of a door with the handle missing). They also take longer than unimpaired readers to name pictures of everyday objects such as a table, car, or window. These differences must be treated with caution however, as instead of reflecting difficulties with processing the visual image, they may actually reflect difficulties with language, i.e. producing the name that is associated with the picture.

In one study that compared dyslexic readers' ability to identify visual signs and symbols without requiring the naming of those symbols, Gregory Brachacki and colleagues at Sheffield University showed individuals a series of genuine road traffic signs and false traffic signs. These false signs were designed to look similar to the genuine signs – a symbol from a genuine sign might be presented on the background of a different-shaped or different-coloured sign, or a critical element of a sign might be deleted or altered in some way. Dyslexic and non-dyslexic readers were shown these signs one at a time on a computer screen and asked to press a button as quickly as possible if they thought the signs were genuine. Dyslexic readers were much poorer at identifying genuine traffic signs than were the non-dyslexic readers. Furthermore, while the performance of the non-dyslexic readers depended on their driving experience – those who had been driving for longer were much better on this task than were those who had been driving for a shorter period of time – no such effect was found for the dyslexic readers.

In an interesting twist on this study, Hermundur Sigmundsson at the Norwegian University of Science and Technology employed a real world driving task to test dyslexic readers' visual-processing skills – their ability to notice, and to respond quickly to, a road sign – whilst operating a driving simulator. Participants in this study sat in a model car and were asked to control the position of the car relative to a car in front, displayed on a video screen. While controlling their virtual car, individuals were asked to press a button or speak aloud when a road sign appeared. Dyslexic readers responded on average 0.19 seconds (30%) slower to the appearance of the road signs than did the non-dyslexic readers. While this difference doesn't sound that great, it would correspond to a distance of 4.4 metres for a car travelling at eighty kilometres (fifty miles) per hour.

These findings suggest that the process of driving – controlling the speed and position of a car, and keeping a watch on the changing traffic situation – takes up most of the dyslexic driver's attention, so they have little spare attention for performing a second task at the same time, in this case watching out for road signs. The study's author did point out, however, that these findings should not be interpreted as suggesting that dyslexic readers are poorer drivers than are non-dyslexic readers, just that the process of driving is less automatic for dyslexic drivers than it is for non-dyslexic ones.

An alternative explanation for these findings might be that dyslexic readers' slower response to the appearance of road signs might reflect a greater difficulty with the processing of rapidly changing visual information. This is similar to the difficulties that dyslexic readers have with processing rapidly changing sounds that were described in chapter 3. This idea supports a hypothesis put forward by some that visual-perceptual problems may be at a more fundamental level, in the functioning of the visual system. The visual system is the neural pathway in the brain which carries visual information from the retina in the eye to the visual cortex at the back of the brain.

Within this system are different clusters of cells whose job it is to detect the orientation, movement, direction, and depth of visual stimuli. If these cells fail to work as they should then the individual will experience visual processing problems. They will have difficulty bringing the eyes to converge steadily on a single spot (known as poor binocular convergence), have difficulty

focusing the eyes (poor fixation stability), and experience difficulty following a moving target (poor visual tracking).

In one test of this, dyslexic readers were found to be poorer
than non-dyslexic readers at detecting clusters of dots on a
computer screen that moved *en masse*, in the same direction and
at the same speed, against a background of randomly moving
dots. The dyslexic readers generally needed to see a larger cluster
of coherently moving dots than did unimpaired readers before
they could detect them.

Dyslexic readers have also been shown to be poorer and
slower than non-dyslexic readers on tasks in which they are
asked to analyse rapidly presented visual information. For
example, to locate a target symbol such as:

//

that is presented for a very brief time surrounded by similar,
distracter symbols such as:

||

For dyslexic readers, the symbols need to be visible for a longer
period of time for them to be located.

The presence of abnormally functioning cells in the visual
system, and the visual-perceptual difficulties that they cause,
might explain why printed text appears to be blurry and to move
around on the page, and why someone might have difficulty
keeping their place as their eyes scan a page of text. However,
while these visual difficulties are more commonly reported in
dyslexic readers than in non-dyslexic readers, they are not exclusively associated with dyslexia.

Eyeballs, rods, and essential fatty acids

Some researchers have attempted to explain visual processing
difficulties in dyslexia in terms of the functioning of the eyeballs.

The inner surface of the back of the eyes, the retina, contains over 130 million cells called photoreceptors. These detect light and convert it into signals that the brain is able to process. There are two types of photoreceptors: rod cells (numbering approximately 125 million) and cone cells (approximately six million). Cone cells function in bright light and enable us to see colour; they are found mainly in and around the centre of the retina, a region called the fovea. Rod cells are particularly sensitive to light and enable us to see in dim light; they are found mainly around the outer edges of the retina.

When we look forwards, everything that we can see without moving our eyes, from the furthest point to our left to the further point to our right, from the furthest point above us to the furthest point below us, falls within what is called our visual field. Visual information that falls on the fovea is sharply focused. The brightness and colour of this part of the visual image are detected by the high concentrations of cone cells within the fovea. Everything else within the visual field – information that falls around the outer edges of the retina, beyond the fovea – is seen in less sharp focus and in less clear colour because rod cells are poor at detecting colour.

Although this issue is rather contentious, it has been suggested that the eyes of dyslexic and non-dyslexic readers have a different pattern of distribution of rod cells and cone cells. Some researchers have indicated that cone cells have a wider distribution in the eyes of dyslexic readers than in the eyes of unimpaired readers. That is, in dyslexic readers' eyes, cone cells appear not only in the fovea but also around the outer edges of the retina. This has the effect that dyslexic readers are better able to identify letters and colours that are presented at the edges of the visual field while non-dyslexic readers are better able to identify letters that are presented in the centre of the visual field. However, there is currently not much evidence to support this suggestion that rod cells and cone cells differ in their distribution in dyslexic and non-dyslexic readers' eyes.

One idea that has received rather more support (anecdotal, if not necessarily scientific) is based on reports that some dyslexic readers have particularly poor night vision and slow dark adaptation, i.e. when they go from a brightly lit room to a darkened room it takes a long time for their vision to adjust so that they are able to see. This has been explained in terms of impaired functioning of the rod cells, itself attributable to a deficiency in essential fatty acids. Rod cells need high concentrations of fatty acids to enable them to function properly but these acids cannot be produced by the body. Instead they must come from the individual's diet, most commonly from fish oils and evening primrose oil. So is it possible that the poor night vision of these dyslexic readers may result from a dietary deficiency of these oils? In support of this proposed link between fatty acid deficiency and dyslexia, some research has shown that people with the greatest fatty acid deficiency are also those who have the greatest number of dyslexia 'symptoms' and the poorest reading and spelling.

A small number of rather high-profile studies have attempted to demonstrate improvements in dark adaptation and reading performance in individuals following a course of fatty acid supplements (omega-3 and omega-6 fatty acids, and vitamin E). These studies are fraught with methodological problems, however, not least:

1. the small numbers of individuals involved;
2. the short periods over which supplements are administered;
3. the consistent absence of a control group. In scientific trials, a control group is treated in exactly the same way as the experimental group except that they do not receive the drug or treatment that is being tested. Researchers compare the performance of the two groups after a period of time to

examine the effects of the drug or treatment. This is the only way of determining that any changes in performance of the experimental group are due to the drug or treatment and not to any other factors. None of these fatty acid trials have included a control group so it is not possible to conclude that improvements in reading and spelling ability in the children who received the supplements are the result of ingesting the fatty acids.

Furthermore, there is a need to show that individuals in these trials are free from attention deficit/hyperactivity disorder (ADHD) which often occurs alongside dyslexia. ADHD has also been associated with fatty acid deficiency. Any improvements in reading ability in individuals with both dyslexia and ADHD may only reflect the reduction of ADHD symptoms following fatty acid supplementation, which would enhance the individual's ability to concentrate and to learn, rather than any possible *treatment* of the dyslexia.

Seeing the world through rose-tinted lenses

As well as having problems with adapting to poor light, and words refusing to stay still on the paper, some dyslexic readers (around 35–40%) also experience visual stress (or glare) from reading black text against a white background; this may be printed text on paper, writing on a whiteboard, or text on a computer screen. This problem is exacerbated by sitting in a room lit by fluorescent lighting. Individuals who experience such problems – not all dyslexic readers do, and not all who experience these problems are dyslexic – are described as having light sensitivity. This is also sometimes referred to as scotopic sensitivity syndrome or Meares–Irlen syndrome. This sensitivity is associated with eye strain, sore eyes, and migraine headaches. A dyslexic reader called Robert recalls the difficulties he experienced in his job producing architectural graphics:

> [I] enjoyed that work, but had to wear sunglasses to avoid headaches caused by the combination of fluorescent lights and the whiteness of [the] drawing board.
>
> *Dyslexia, the Self and Higher Education* by David Pollak, p. 130

Research has shown that this visual sensitivity can be reduced by wearing coloured lenses or putting plastic overlays over the page. These measures reduce the glare of the white background and the contrast of the black on white text. Lenses and overlays come in many different colours so the individual can choose the colour that best works for them. The beneficial effects of these lenses and overlays are described by a forty-one-year-old dyslexic man who returned to college as a mature student:

> I had an appointment with … the support tutor for the college … she said, 'take this piece of acetate, this blue stuff … does that make [your reading] any easier?' and it was like somebody had switched the light on in the room! I thought 'this is amazing! What's happened?' you know. And so we went through all these different colours, and I came up with the blue one. So I was carrying these little plastic sheets around, and I found out I have a problem with black on white, especially bright white.
>
> *Dyslexia, the Self and Higher Education* by David Pollak, p. 199

Similarly, dyslexia-friendly websites (e.g. www.bdadyslexia. org.uk) allow individuals to adjust the background colour of webpages – and usually the font colour and size too – to avoid this difficulty with high-contrast (usually black on white) glare from the screen.

While lenses and overlays can improve reading speed and accuracy in some people, particularly if the text is small with closely spaced lines, they don't work for everyone. Only a minority of dyslexic readers experience the visual glare and 'swimming' text that these lenses and overlays are designed to reduce, and not all of those who experience these visual problems find that their reading improves with the use of coloured lenses and overlays.

Dyslexia and eye movements

As we read, our eyes scan across the printed text in a series of rapid step-like movements called *saccades*. These are interspersed with brief periods of fixation, when the eyes stop on a portion of the text, during which we actually process the text. Each fixation occurs for approximately 250 milliseconds, although this time can be longer or shorter depending on the nature and complexity of the text. Familiar words and function words, such as *the*, *and*, *of*, tend to be moved over quite quickly, while we tend to fixate for longer on unfamiliar words and content words, such as *jump*, *lark*, *box*. For example, read the following text:

I love Paris in the
the spring time

You probably failed to notice the superfluous second 'the' in this sentence, at the start of the second line, as your eyes moved across the words. We often skim over function words while still being able to process and understand what we read.

The duration of fixations is also influenced by the ease with which we are able to process the text. While good readers move their eyes in a generally forward direction (left-to-right or right-to-left, depending on the language), dyslexic, poor, and inexperienced readers tend to spend more time looking back over previously read words, making 'regressive saccades'. They also show more frequent fixations that are longer in duration. Some have suggested that these erratic eye movements may cause the reading difficulties of dyslexic readers, although it is rather more likely that they merely reflect the difficulties that these readers experience during reading. Dyslexic, poor, and inexperienced readers spend longer looking at words, and they look back over previously read words, because they are having difficulty reading the words.

Reading weaknesses, visual strengths?

Despite reports of visual-perceptual difficulty in dyslexia, anecdotal evidence has associated dyslexia with superior visuospatial performance. Dyslexia tends to be over-represented, for example, in professions and academic disciplines related to art and design, and many artists and designers credit their dyslexia with helping them to realise their artistic potential. Internationally renowned, and award-winning, furniture and product designer Sebastian Bergne, for example, said:

> When you have choices, you go for what you're good at. If one part of your development is 'blocked', you develop other parts more fully. As a child I got used to expressing things in a different way to writing. I think visually. I think in pictures. If I'm designing an object, I know the exact shape in 3D. I can walk around it in my head before drawing it.

Photographer David Bailey observed:

> I feel dyslexia gave me a privilege. It pushed me into being totally visual.

While John Mishler, whose metal sculptures have been installed in many towns and cities across America, said:

> Being dyslexic has given me an enhanced imagination ... in my head I see visual images that are often turned into sculptures without any drawings on paper. It took me a long time to realise that being dyslexic was a gift.

If dyslexia is accompanied by superior visuospatial ability then it should be found in higher than expected numbers of artists, scientists, and architects who are at the top of their professions. The ten most popular/successful members of these professions are listed in Table 2.

Of the ten most popular artists (at www.artcyclopedia.com/mostpopular.html, based on the number of searches made on the website), four are thought to be dyslexic (these are indicated in the table by an asterisk). So too is Robert Rauschenberg, described by some as 'the greatest living painter'.

Five of the top ten scientists (from the book *The Scientific 100: A Ranking of the Most Influential Scientists, Past and Present* by John Galbraith Simmons) are believed to be dyslexic, as are four of the ten most recent winners of the Pritzker Architecture Prize, colloquially referred to as 'the Nobel prize of architecture'. The most recent recipient of this award, Sir Richard Rogers (also dyslexic), believes strongly in the need to explore the strengths, as well as the weaknesses, of dyslexic readers:

> Dyslexics do have many hurdles to overcome and we do need practical strategies. But after 100 years, it is time to look not only at the difficulties, but at the abilities and the potential that many dyslexic people have.

One ability seems to be visuospatial. Around 40–50% of these eminent artists, architects, and scientists are dyslexic, which is significantly greater than the 5–10% incidence of dyslexia found

Table 2 The ten most successful/popular artists, scientists, and architects

Artists	Scientists	Architects
1. Pablo Picasso★	Isaac Newton★	Richard Rogers★ – Pompidou Centre, Paris; European Court of Human Rights, Strasbourg
2. Vincent van Gogh★	Albert Einstein★	Paulo Mendes da Rocha – FIESP Cultural Center, São Paulo, Brazil
3. Leonardo da Vinci★	Niels Bohr★	Thom Mayne★ – Sun Tower, Seoul, Korea
4. Claude Monet	Charles Darwin★	Zaha Hadid – Rosenthal Center for Contemporary Art, Ohio
5. Andy Warhol★	Louis Pasteur★	Jørn Utzon★ – Sydney Opera House, Australia; National Assembly of Kuwait, Kuwait City
6. Salvador Dali	Sigmund Freud	Glenn Murcutt – Magney House and Done House, Sydney, Australia
7. Georgia O'Keeffe	Galileo Galilei	Jacques Herzog – Tate Modern Art Gallery, London
8. Henri Matisse	Antoine Lavoisier	Rem Koolhaas – Guggenheim Hermitage Museum, Las Vegas
9. Wassily Kandinsky	Johannes Kepler	Norman Foster★ – Hearst Tower, New York City; Wembley Stadium, London
10. Nan Goldin	Nicolaus Copernicus	Renzo Piano – New York Times Building, New York City; Kansai International Airport, Japan

Key: ★Individuals either known to be, or believed to have been, dyslexic in the general population. However, in searching for well-known exemplars of artistic/creative dyslexics, there is a danger that as you seek, so shall you find. Many of the greatest artists, architects and scientists may well be dyslexic but there are many more who are not.

Rather more persuasive may be reports of the number of dyslexic individuals (as a percentage of the student population) studying at various prestigious art colleges in England: 10% at the Surrey Institute of Art and Design; 15% at Central St Martins College of Art and Design in London (this rose to over 30% for foundation students with 'dyslexia-type learning difficulties'); and 25% at London's Royal College of Art. It should be noted that students only gain entry to these art schools on merit not because other, language-based, paths are blocked to them. The author, Beverly Steffert, notes:

> while most art and design students display strong visuospatial abilities, the most innovative students were often those with dyslexia.

In a series of experiments exploring spatial talent in dyslexic adults, Ellen Winner and her research group in Boston found that dyslexic readers out-performed unimpaired readers when they were asked to indicate whether objects drawn in two dimensions could exist in three dimensions. All of the objects looked plausible on close inspection of their individual parts. Viewing each figure as a whole object, however, showed that some could not exist in the real-world – i.e. they were *impossible* figures. Some examples of impossible figures are shown in figure 4.

Dyslexic readers were faster than, but just as accurate as, non-dyslexic readers at recognising the impossibility of these figures. To do this, they needed to take a *global* (holistic) rather than a *local* (analytical) perspective of the images. This ability to take an overview of objects, to see things as wholes, is the skill that the

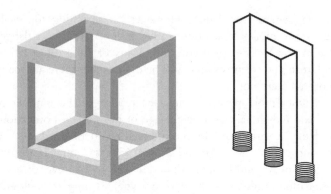

Figure 4 Some 'impossible' figures

authors identified as being necessary for professions such as art, engineering, and architecture, in which dyslexic readers excel.

Support for this idea is provided by research by Neil Martin and myself in which we asked dyslexic and non-dyslexic adults to:

- identify objects in an ambiguous figure – e.g. a drawing that if looked at one way can be seen as a duck, while if looked at another way can be seen as a rabbit;
- recall the direction of the queen's head on a British postage stamp (in case you're not sure, she faces left, towards the address);
- familiarise themselves with a simple, computer-based virtual reality town and then recreate the town using scale cardboard models of the buildings and a plan with the roads drawn on; credit was given for showing the correct locations of the buildings relative to the town's roads and to each other.

Dyslexic men were more accurate than dyslexic women and unimpaired readers on the ambiguous figures task, and at recalling the direction of the queen's head on a stamp. Dyslexic men were also faster and more accurate than dyslexic women and unimpaired men at recreating the virtual reality town.

If some dyslexic readers genuinely possess superior, holistic visuospatial ability, then those who enter, and excel in, visuo-spatial and creative professions might demonstrate this ability in their work. Notable examples of this exist in the form of award-winning lighting and furniture designer, Terence Woodgate, who observes that:

> Visualisation is one of my strengths as a designer. I think I'm particularly good with mechanisms. I can see the whole thing finished and working. I don't need paper. I like to design while driving or showering. I'm sure this is because part of my brain is distracted, leaving the creative side to dream. It's as though we dyslexics have a 3D graphics card integrated into our heads.

And John Chambers, President and CEO of Cisco Systems (the company that develops routers and software – the 'plumbing' – for the internet), who told Fortune Magazine in 2002:

> I can't explain why, but I just approach problems differently ... I picture a chess game on a multiple-layer dimensional cycle and almost play it out in my mind ... I don't make moves one at a time. I can usually anticipate the potential outcome and where the Ys in the road will occur. I'm very good at seeing something and memorizing the whole concept.

In the same article, biologist and inventor Bill Dreyer (whose invention of a protein-sequencing machine enabled the launch of the human genome project) expressed a similar idea as he explained the way his mind works:

> I was able to see the machine in my head and rotate valves and actually see the instrumentation ... I think in 3-D Technicolor pictures instead of words. I don't think of dyslexia as a deficiency. It's like having CAD [computer-aided design] in your brain.

If these artists, engineers, architects, and inventors are right, how might the relationship between dyslexia and superior visuo-spatial ability be explained? There are three possible explanations:

1. It could be a specious correlation.

   There should be just as many visuospatially talented dyslexic readers as visuospatially talented non-dyslexic readers. While non-dyslexic readers with spatial talents might be as likely to choose an occupation that demands verbal or spatial abilities, dyslexic readers with spatial talents would not have the luxury of this choice. This would explain the disproportionate number of dyslexic readers in visuospatial fields, but not a general difference between the spatial abilities of dyslexic and non-dyslexic readers.

2. It could reflect a 'pathology of superiority'.

   The neurologist Norman Geschwind suggested that dyslexia is associated with a 'pathology of superiority', where the right side of the brain (which is associated with holistic, spatial processing) is more developed than normal because of poor development of the linguistic, left side of the brain. This has been seen post-mortem in four adult, male dyslexic readers (who are described in chapter 6). Of these four, in life one had been a skilled metal sculptor, one a qualified engineer, and one was 'athletically gifted'.

3. It could reflect a dyslexic processing strategy.

   Dyslexic readers may preferentially adopt a visuospatial processing style rather than a verbal processing style. That is, they may tend to solve problems by creating mental images of the problems rather than by thinking through the problems using words. Such a difference has been found when dyslexic and non-dyslexic readers solve syllogisms – a form of deductive reasoning consisting of:

   a. a major premise, such as 'All swans are white';
   b a minor premise, 'This bird is white'; and
   c. a conclusion, 'This bird is a swan'.

Assuming that the major and minor premises are true, the task is to decide whether the conclusion is also necessarily true. Dyslexic men and women are more likely to adopt a visuospatial reasoning strategy when solving syllogisms. For example, they will draw simple Venn diagrams, with overlapping circles representing each premise. Non-dyslexic readers are more likely to adopt a verbal strategy by thinking through the possible relationships between the groups described in each premise.

There may be some merit in all three of these explanations although further research is needed to determine the extent to which each one is able to explain the apparent relationship between dyslexia and superior visuospatial ability. One strand of this research is described next.

Dyslexia and learning styles

Since the late 1990s some considerable interest has been taken in learning styles, and the possible existence of a *dyslexic learning style* in particular. The term learning style refers to someone's usual, and preferred, way of processing information. This is generally determined through responses to items on a questionnaire; there are many to choose from. Someone may be identified as having a certain learning style or falling somewhere on a continuum between two styles. Unfortunately, researchers disagree on the number and type of learning styles that people in general may have. Possible styles range from:

- a preference for thinking in words (verbal style) to a preference for thinking in images (visual style);
- a tendency to see the big picture (holistic style) to a tendency to focus on individual details (analytic style);
- a preference for learning by seeing how to do things (visual learning) to learning by being told how to do things

(auditory learning) or learning by doing thing 'hands-on' (kinaesthetic learning);
- learning by analysing facts (assimilative learning) to learning by trial and error (accommodative learning);
- learning by doing (impulsive learning) to learning by thinking (reflective learning).

Some have suggested that the characteristic dyslexic learning style is predominantly visual, holistic, kinaesthetic, accommodative, and impulsive. We all learn most effectively when we are taught to our strengths rather than to our weaknesses. Dyslexic readers should learn best by seeing and doing; by visualising words, spellings, and problems as complete units; they should learn by seeing patterns within words, and by being given the chance to practice (even over-practice) until a skill is acquired. This approach underlies the multi-sensory teaching method, described in chapter 8, that is increasingly being used with dyslexic readers. However, this way of learning may be a far more general learning style than a dyslexic learning style. Evidence from the classroom suggests that most children, whether dyslexic or non-dyslexic, benefit from this method of teaching.

Dyslexia is no longer considered to be purely a problem of visual perception, although many dyslexic readers experience subtle visual difficulties caused by abnormal functioning of the cells in the visual system. Many dyslexic readers also excel in professions and academic disciplines related to art and design although the reason for this is currently unclear. The next chapter considers the importance of visual processing and phonological processing for reading and dyslexia in different alphabetic and non-alphabetic languages.

Is dyslexia universal?

AS was born in Japan to a highly literate Australian father and English mother, and goes to a Japanese selective senior high school in Japan. His spoken language at home is English. AS's reading in Japanese Kanji and Kana is equivalent to that of Japanese undergraduates or graduates. In contrast, his performance in various reading and writing tests in English as well as tasks involving phonological processing was very poor, even when compared to his Japanese contemporaries … AS is severely dyslexic in just one of his languages [English]. In the other [Japanese], he performs at a superior level.

Wydell and Butterworth (1999)

One aspect of a language that determines how easy or difficult it is to learn to read is its regularity. The regularity of a language is the consistency of the relationship between the written letters and their spoken sounds. Regular languages, where written letters consistently map onto their spoken sounds, are said to have a *shallow*, or *transparent*, orthography (relationship between written letters and their sounds). Irregular languages are said to have a *deep*, or *opaque*, orthography. Table 3 illustrates some languages with deep and shallow orthographies.

Languages such as Italian, Finnish and Spanish are highly regular. They have a consistent mapping between written letters and their spoken sounds, and so are identified as having a shallow orthography. The spelling rules of these languages are straightforward and easy to learn. The ultimate example of a regular language seems to be Serbo-Croatian, which is perfectly

Table 3 Some deep and shallow alphabetic languages

Deep (irregular) languages			←————————→	Shallow (regular) languages	
English	Danish	Dutch	Gaelic	Finnish	
	French	Portuguese	German	Serbo-Croatian	
		Swedish	Greek		
			Hungarian		
			Icelandic		
			Italian		
			Norwegian		
			Spanish		
			Turkish		
			Welsh		

transparent. Each of the thirty-three individual written letters can only be pronounced in one way, and each spoken sound can only be written in one way. Italian readers are also fortunate in that they only need to learn thirty-three letters/letter combinations to represent the twenty-five sounds that make up their language. Novice readers of the language, once they are familiar with the fundamental spelling-sound rules, are soon able to read Italian text accurately.

By contrast, languages such as English, Danish, and French are irregular. They have a complex mapping between written letters and their spoken sounds, and so are identified as having a deep orthography. The spelling rules of these languages are ambiguous and difficult to learn. In English, this involves the often ambiguous mapping of 1,120 letters/letter combinations onto the forty sounds that make up the spoken language. Consider, for example, the following peculiarities of the language:

- the different pronunciations of the word pairs *mint/pint*, *dive/live*, and *gave/have*;

- the number of ways in which the letter sequence 'ough' can be pronounced, e.g. in *cough*, *hiccough*, *bough*, *through*, *thought*;
- the number of ways in which the spoken 'k' sound can be represented, e.g. by the single letter 'k' (as in *walk*), by the single letter 'c' (as in *stoical*), by the letters 'cc' (as in *raccoon*), by the letters 'ch' (as in *school*), and the letters 'ck' (as in *trick*)

and you'll appreciate why English spelling has been described as 'the world's most awesome mess'.

Try using your knowledge of English rules of pronunciation to help you to read this made-up word: ghoti. Say it out loud. Now think about the pronunciation of the letters 'gh' as in the word *cough*. Keep this sound ('f') in the back of your mind. Next, think about the pronunciation of the letter 'o' in the word *women* ('i') and add this onto the 'f'. Finally, think about the pronunciation of the letters 'ti' in *station* and add this 'sh' sound onto the end of the previous sounds. Does this pronunciation ('fish') in any way resemble your earlier attempt at reading the word *ghoti*?

A similar example is the surname *Featherstonehaugh* which, by some bizarre, historical quirk of the English language is pronounced as 'Fan'-'shaw'. Such is the joy of English that the spelling of an unfamiliar word cannot be relied upon to tell us how to pronounce it. Little wonder then that so many foreign tourists (even English-speaking ones) are thrown into confusion by place names in Great Britain, such as Leicester (pronounced 'Le'-'ster'), Alcester ('Ol'-'ster') or Edinburgh ('Edin'-'bu'-'ruh'), or places in America, such as Arkansas ('Ark'-'in'-'saw'), Des Moines ('De'-'moyne') or Sequim ('Skwim'). Don't be lulled into a false sense of security by place names that are common to both countries. Different possible pronunciations of the same string of letters have led to identically written place names, such as Leominster, being pronounced in different ways in the UK (where it is pronounced 'Lem'-'ster') and in the US (where it is pronounced 'Lem'-'en'-'ster').

Learning to read in shallow and deep orthographies

Unsurprisingly, the regularity of a language has a direct bearing on how children learn to read. Children whose native language is shallow should be able to learn to read and spell much more rapidly and easily than those whose native language is deep. A large, cross-language research project comparing the development of letter knowledge and the reading of simple words and non-words in six- to seven-year-old children, from thirteen European countries supported this theory (see www.dundee.ac.uk/psychology/collesrc/welcome.htm for more details). This project found that reading accuracy by the end of the first year of school was:

- almost 100% in Finnish-, Greek-, and German-speaking children;
- around 92–95% for speakers of Italian, Spanish, Swedish, Dutch, Icelandic, and Norwegian;
- around 70–80% for speakers of French, Portuguese, and Danish; and
- around 34% for English-speaking children.

Similar findings also emerge for the reading of non-words. Measuring a child's ability to read non-words may seen nonsensical, but actually provides an accurate measure of a child's ability to understand the spelling-sound rules of the language. These non-words are unfamiliar so must be decoded letter-by-letter, they cannot be recognised as whole words.

By the end of the first year of school around 90–95% of Norwegian-, Finnish-, Greek-, and German-speaking children could read non-words accurately. So could:

- around 82–89% of Italian, Spanish, Swedish, Dutch, Icelandic, and French children;
- 77% of Portuguese children;
- 54% of Danish children; and
- 29% of English-speaking children.

Even by the end of the second year at school English children are only able to read around 45% of non-words. This shows that the development of foundation literacy skills in English-speaking children occurs twice as slowly as in non-English-speaking European children.

The results mirror what we would predict on the basis of the regularity of the languages. Children whose native languages are irregular and inconsistent experience much greater difficulty learning the spelling-sound rules of their languages than do children whose native languages are regular and consistent. This is reflected in the accuracy of non-word reading across the thirteen languages, and particularly in the English-speakers.

In the UK and the USA children start attending school from the age of five, or sometimes shortly before their fifth birthday, and immediately begin to receive reading instruction. This builds upon basic literacy skills that they have learned in their pre-school years. This is in contrast to children from other countries, particularly the Scandinavian countries, such as Finland and Norway, who typically do not begin formal reading instruction until the age of six or seven. So the results reported above – accuracy for the reading of words and non-words – are actually comparing children of different ages. The English-speaking children are often one or two years younger than the non-English-speaking children. Even so, the English children's reading accuracy after two years at school, by which time they are seven years old, is still considerably poorer than that of the other seven-year-old children at the end of their first year at school.

The good news is that while the English-speaking children are considerably slower at developing these early literacy skills than are their non-English-speaking counterparts, they do catch up. While seven-year-old Finnish children are able to read with 90% accuracy after around ten weeks of reading instruction in school, English-speaking children may take four or five years to achieve this same level of reading accuracy. Differences in the reading ability of speakers of different languages have generally disappeared by the time the children reach the age of eleven or twelve years.

The orthographic depth hypothesis – the strong version

To explain differences in reading accuracy between readers of different languages, researchers have proposed the *orthographic depth hypothesis*. This suggests that languages that differ in the complexity (or depth) of their spelling-sound rules are read in different ways, i.e. by following different paths through the dual route model of reading that we looked at in chapter 2.

Speakers of relatively shallow languages should always rely on a phonological route from print to sound by breaking words down into their constituent sounds. Since these languages have a consistent relationship between written letters/letter clusters and their pronunciations, individuals should be able to achieve 100% reading accuracy of all words and non-words by follow-ing the sub-lexical, phonological route as they read. Readers of shallow languages would have no need to access a mental word list (lexicon) to achieve reading accuracy.

By contrast, speakers of relatively deep languages are unable to rely solely on a phonological route from print to sound if they are to read irregular words and non-words accurately. These readers are better served by reading via the lexical route: whole words are 'looked up' in the mental lexicon and their meanings and pronunciations are obtained.

However, research does not entirely support this hypothesis. Speakers of shallow languages do have to access the mental lexicon in their reading to provide them with information regarding the stress patterns of words – i.e. which syllable within a word should be stressed. To provide examples from English:

- The word *envelope* is stressed on the first syllable.
- The word *tomato* is stressed on the second syllable.
- The word *volunteer* is stressed on the third syllable.

This information is not available via the phonological route yet some of the most consistent, regular languages have inconsistent, and unpredictable, stress patterns. In Italian, for example, stress is placed in the following way:

- on the last syllable in approximately 4% of words – e.g. *leggerò*, meaning 'I will read';
- on the second-to-last syllable in approximately 84% of words. This is the most regular (common) stress pattern in Italian – e.g. *leggere*, meaning 'light'; and
- on the third-to-last syllable in approximately 12% of words – e.g. *leggere*, meaning 'to read'.

The importance of the mental lexicon to Italian is also illustrated by reports of Italian stroke patients who have suffered damage to the language areas of their brains. These patients are still able to read around 98% of non-words and regularly stressed real words (those that are stressed on the second-to-last syllable) accurately. Their ability to read words that are stressed irregularly (on the third-to-last or last syllables), however, drops to around 79%. These findings have been interpreted as showing that the regular stress pattern (with stress placed on the second-to-last syllable) is assigned by default unless information to the contrary is stored in the lexicon. Italian patients with damage to their lexicon will, therefore, tend to produce regular stress patterns for words by default. Of course, in most cases this will be correct.

Readers of both shallow and deep languages demonstrate what are called *lexical priming effects*. In lexical priming experiments, individuals are asked to read words that are selected to 'prime' (prompt) the reading of subsequent words. Words may be primed visually, such that reading the word *peak* may prime the reading of the word *beak*, or semantically, such that reading the word *bread* may prime the reading of the word *butter*. Following this priming the individual is likely to read the second word faster than they would have done if the word had not been primed. This effect has been observed in several shallow languages including Spanish, Dutch, Serbo-Croatian, and Italian, as well as English, suggesting that these readers are all reading by 'looking words up' in the mental lexicon. In the mental lexicon words that are in some way related – i.e. they are commonly used together, such as *table* and *chair* or *mouse* and *cheese* – are linked. If the readers of these shallow languages were relying solely on phonological letter-sound translation, this lexical priming effect would not be found.

The orthographic depth hypothesis – the weak version

A 'weaker' version of the orthographic depth hypothesis suggests that reading in all languages, deep or shallow, involves both phonological and lexical processes. The difference between deep and shallow languages is seen in the *extent* to which readers rely on phonological and lexical processes. Readers of shallow languages are more likely to rely on phonological processes for reading, while readers of deep languages are more likely to rely on lexical processes.

Evidence for this is provided by research showing that young readers of shallow languages (German, Welsh, Spanish, Italian, and Greek) are more accurate at reading non-words (which must be read via a phonological route) than are readers of deep languages (English or French). Readers of shallow languages are also more likely than readers of deep languages to accept that pseudo-homophones are real words; pseudo-homophones are made-up words that are created to sound like real words without looking like them, e.g. 'focks' or 'dore'. This indicates that these shallow readers are relying, to a greater extent than deep readers, on a phonological reading strategy.

A collaborative study between researchers at University College London and the University of Milan-Bicocca compared English and Italian adults' reading of high-frequency (common) regular words from their native language (e.g. *cabin*, *market*, *cottage*; *marmo*, *ponte*, *moto*), non-words based on these words (e.g. *cagin*, *marnet*, *connage*; *margo*, *ponda*, *moco*), and familiar 'international' words that have the same spelling and meaning in both languages. Half of these international words conformed to English spelling patterns, the other half to Italian patterns. The 'English' words, *partner*, *basket*, *corner*, for example, contain clusters of consonants that do not appear in Italian (e.g. the 'rtn' in *partner*), the letter 'k', which is rare in Italian and only appears in words of foreign derivation, and all of the words end in consonants (most Italian words end in vowels). The 'Italian' words, such as *coma*, *villa*, *pasta*, all end in vowels (which is far rarer in English) and unlike English words, their letters are consistently pronounced.

In this study, the Italian students were consistently faster reading the Italian real words and non-words than the English students were reading the English words and non-words. This finding has been labelled by Uta Frith, one of the study's authors, as 'the Ferrari effect' (referring to the speed of the Italian sports cars and the speed of the Italian readers). Both groups read real words faster than they read non-words although this difference was greater for the English students.

An interesting finding emerged for the reading of the international words in that the Italian readers were faster reading words that conformed to their own rules of spelling than those that conformed to the English rules. No such effect emerged for the English readers. Brain imaging data gathered from the same study showed more activity in the English readers' brains, during reading, in regions associated with whole word reading/picture naming. Italian readers' brains showed more activity in a region associated with phonological processing. These results provide further support for the weak version of the orthographic depth hypothesis.

The grain size theory

In a slight modification of the orthographic depth hypotheses, the grain size theory proposes that while reading in any language entails converting spelling into sound, the size of the letter strings – the 'grain size' – into which words are broken down depends on the depth of the language. In shallow languages, in which single letters consistently represent single sounds, the grain size is very small. Therefore, children quickly learn that words can be read on a letter-by-letter basis. In deep languages children cannot rely solely on letter-by-letter reading if they are to avoid making frequent reading errors. Instead, these children need to learn how to convert strings of letters with a larger grain size (e.g. 'alk', 'ough', 'tion') into their corresponding sounds to enable them to read efficiently and accurately.

In support of this theory, German readers' reading of words and non-words seems to be predominantly influenced by the number of letters in the words/non-words whereas English readers' reading seems to be influenced by the structure of the words or non-words. German readers' reading of non-words is helped when the non-words share letters with familiar real words. For example, the non-word *loffee*, that shares the majority of its letters with the word *toffee*, is read faster than the non-word *pontle* that bears little visual resemblance to any real words. Similarly, English readers read non-words that sound like real words (e.g. *faik*) more quickly than they read ones that do not (e.g. *daik*), while German readers show no such difference. These findings suggest that whereas German readers employ efficient small-grain, letter-by-letter reading, English readers tend to employ a reading strategy that is based on a larger grain size, even up to the level of the whole word.

Unlike some of its predecessors, the grain size theory of reading is able to explain the development of different reading strategies in deep and shallow languages. It also explains differences in the incidence of dyslexia across languages, the topic of the next section.

Dyslexia across different languages

As you have seen so far, the ease with which children learn to read and spell depends, to a large extent, on their native language. It should come as no surprise that the estimated incidence of developmental dyslexia also depends on the depth of the language. Estimates of the incidence of dyslexia range between 5% and 15% for speakers of alphabetic languages, although this figure masks some quite striking differences in the incidence of dyslexia across different languages (illustrated in figure 5).

Note that the languages in this figure are divided by their orthographic depth, with the deep languages (Chinese, Danish, and English) at the top and the shallow languages at the bottom of the figure. There is a fairly clear distinction, with only one or two exceptions, between the incidence of dyslexia in the

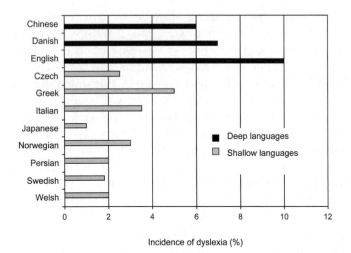

Figure 5 The estimated incidence of dyslexia across different languages

shallow and deep languages. However, this picture is muddled by the fact that countries differ in the way they describe dyslexia. In some there is generally poor understanding of what dyslexia is and how it manifests itself. Some have no official, standardised definition at all. Even in the United States, different states have their own particular definitions of dyslexia. Other countries use 'dyslexia' as a general catch-all term that includes other, more general, learning difficulties. In view of these differences in the definition and description of dyslexia, it is difficult to compare the true incidence of dyslexia across countries. It is agreed, however, that the phonological difficulties of dyslexia are universal. The extent to which these difficulties impede the reading development of children in different countries depends on the depth of the language spoken in those countries.

Dyslexia in deep and shallow languages

While dyslexic readers of all languages have difficulty converting written letters into their corresponding sounds, those who need to translate between the spoken and written forms of complex, deep, irregular languages will be the ones who experience the greatest reading difficulty. While these 'deep' readers will display the slow and impaired reading, spelling, and phonological processing that is typical of dyslexia, dyslexic readers of shallow languages may cope adequately with their daily reading; their reading accuracy is likely to be no poorer than that of non-dyslexic readers although their reading will be markedly slower.

Studies of German and English dyslexic readers offer a neat opportunity to compare the abilities of readers of shallow (German) and deep (English) languages using words and non-words that are as similar as possible. As English and German developed from the same Germanic root they share many words in common, such as the German words *Ball, Katze, Salat* and the English equivalents, *ball, cat, salad*. The main difference in the pronunciation of these words lies in the vowels. Whereas the 'a' in each of the German words is pronounced consistently as a short 'a' sound (as in the English word *cat*), the 'a' in each of the English words is pronounced inconsistently, as an 'or' sound in *ball*, as a short 'a' sound in *cat*, and in the word *salad* as a short 'a' followed by an 'u' sound.

While German dyslexic children read the consistent German words with around 97% accuracy, English dyslexic readers of the same age read around 81% of the inconsistent English words accurately. When these children were asked to read infrequent (less commonly used) words accuracy rates dropped to 89% for the German children and 48% for the English children, and when they were asked to read non-words accuracy dropped even further, to 77% for the German children and 27% for the English children.

Because of the consistency of German, reading in Germany and Austria is predominantly taught using phonics-based reading schemes, and children (even dyslexic ones) quickly learn which letters represent which sounds. English-speaking dyslexic children are not so fortunate, however. The inconsistency of their language makes reading high frequency words – which can be mostly recognised by sight – slightly more difficult, while reading low frequency words and non-words – which need to be phonologically recoded – is much more difficult.

While the consistency of the German language allows German-speaking dyslexic readers to develop fairly accurate reading skills, the difficulties of dyslexia manifest in these individuals in other ways, including:

- slow reading speed – dyslexic children's reading is described as being 'painstakingly slow' and laborious, such that twelve-year-old German-speaking dyslexic children read at the same speed as typically developing six- to eight-year-old German readers;
- slow naming of objects, animals, and numbers;
- difficulty deleting sounds from spoken words (e.g. saying *helfen* (*help*) without the 'f'); dyslexic children make around twice as many errors as do non-dyslexic children;
- difficulty repeating multi-syllabic non-words (e.g. *ripschofkut*), demonstrating poor short-term memory.

Other signs of dyslexia in readers of shallow languages may be poor organisation, poor timekeeping, poor sense of direction, difficulty remembering facts, difficulty remembering sequences of instructions, and mispronunciation of some words, such as saying 'busgetti' instead of *spaghetti*.

A cross-language study of English, Italian, and French adults tested the reading and phonological skills of dyslexic and non-dyslexic university students. While the researchers had no difficulty finding English and French dyslexic readers, Italian dyslexic readers were difficult to find. From screening 1,200 Italian students, they were able to identify only eighteen dyslexic readers, and these only on the basis of their extremely slow reading speed. Participants were asked to:

- read real words, such as *window, pocket, carrot*;
- read non-words, such as *wimpow, podret, cassot*;
- listen to pairs of words and repeat the words with the initial sounds swapped around, so the words *basket* and *lemon*, for example, become *lasket* and *bemon*.

The study found that the Italian dyslexic readers were consistently more accurate at reading words and non-words than were either of the other dyslexic samples. All three dyslexic groups were poorer at reading and at swapping the initial sounds between words than were the non-dyslexic groups.

These and other results suggest that English and French, German and Italian dyslexic readers – as well as dyslexic readers of other shallow languages including Spanish, Italian, Dutch, and Czech – experience similar phonological difficulties. These phonological difficulties, as chapter 6 suggests, may have a common brain-based (neuro-anatomical) origin although they manifest themselves in different ways depending on the depth of the language. The combination of phonological difficulties and the inconsistency of deep languages cause dyslexic readers of these languages to read poorly and slowly, while the combination of phonological difficulties and the consistency of shallow languages enables dyslexic readers of these languages to read accurately, albeit slowly.

Phonological processing in dyslexic readers of deep and shallow languages

An interesting finding from studies with dyslexic children has shown that during the first few years of schooling speakers of both shallow and deep languages experience phonological processing difficulties. First and second grade Dutch, Greek, Italian, French, and Austrian dyslexic children have difficulty reading and spelling non-words. Around 97% of first grade Greek unimpaired readers are able to read non-words correctly, but this figure drops to 93% for children with dyslexia. For Austrian children figures of 96% and around 60% are reported. Some researchers have suggested that these difficulties disappear by the end of second grade, by which time the phonological abilities of dyslexic readers have 'caught up' with those of non-dyslexic readers.

German-speaking dyslexic readers from the third grade are virtually perfect at spelling non-words, indicating that they have grasped the fundamental spelling-sound rules of the language. Similarly, while pre-school Dutch dyslexic children are poor at identifying which word out of three does not rhyme with the other two (i.e. they demonstrate simple phonological difficulties), they are able to perform this task by the end of first grade. More difficult tests of phonological awareness, such as identifying which word of three ends in a different sound to the other two (e.g. *hat*, *cat*, *man*, *bat*), are beyond the capabilities of pre-school dyslexic children but they are able to perform this task as well as unimpaired readers by the end of sixth grade. A combination of the shallow German and Dutch orthographies and the use of phonics-based reading instruction seems to enable even phonologically challenged dyslexic readers to overcome their early difficulties.

However, others have found persistent phonological difficulties in speakers of shallow languages beyond the early school years. For example, the word and non-word spelling ability of eleven-year-old Czech dyslexic readers has been analysed and their responses classified as either phonologically accurate or phonologically inaccurate:

- Phonologically accurate spelling represents all the sounds of the word (so it *sounds* correct) even if the word is spelt incorrectly. For example, the word *please* might be spelt as 'please', 'plees', or 'pleez'. All of these responses are phonologically accurate.
- Phonologically inaccurate spelling fails to represent all the sounds of the word. For example, the word *please* might be spelt as 'plays', 'pls', or 'bls'.

Despite the consistency of their language, the dyslexic children produced significantly more phonologically inaccurate spellings than did their non-dyslexic peers such that:

- 19% of the dyslexic children's spelling of words, and 4% of the non-dyslexic children's, were classified as being phonologically inaccurate.
- 28% of the dyslexic children's spelling of non-words, and 7% of the non-dyslexic children's, were classified as being phonologically inaccurate.

Czech dyslexic readers aged seven to twelve years (grades three to seven) are also poorer than unimpaired readers of the same age on tests requiring them to delete the first, second, or third sound from single-syllable words, and to swap the initial sounds of pairs of spoken one-syllable and two-syllable words. Others have found evidence of persistent phonological difficulties in Dutch, French, and Hebrew dyslexic children, at least up to sixth grade, when the phonological task used was sufficiently taxing. For example, requiring children to delete sounds from within two-syllable non-words (e.g. delete the middle sound from the word *memslos*).

Together these findings show that phonological difficulties are a consistent feature of dyslexia across deep and shallow alphabetic languages, at least through the primary school years. The precise nature of these difficulties, however, varies with the depth of the language.

Dyslexic readers of shallow languages may learn to master relatively simple phonological skills, such as recognising and producing rhyme and alliteration, within their first few years at school. More complex phonological skills such as adding, deleting and swapping sounds within and between words take longer to master. As you saw in the study of English, Italian, and French dyslexic adults, Italian dyslexic readers are able to manipulate the sounds of words more efficiently than are either French or English dyslexic readers. The consistency of Italian has enabled them to develop these phonological skills but they are still not as good, or as fast, at doing so as non-dyslexic readers.

By contrast, dyslexic readers of deep languages continue to show poor phonological skills into adulthood. The phonological difficulties that these readers face typically manifest themselves as slow and inaccurate reading (particularly of irregular words, such as *aisle*), inaccurate spelling, and frequent mispronunciation of long words (such as *phenomenal*).

Dyslexia in non-alphabetic languages

So far we have looked exclusively at dyslexia in speakers of alphabetic languages. But what about non-alphabetic languages? Do dyslexic readers of these languages experience the same difficulties as dyslexic readers of alphabetic languages? To understand why they may or indeed, why they may not, let us take a simplified look at two non-alphabetic languages, Chinese and Japanese (including kana and kanji).

A common misconception about the Chinese script is that it

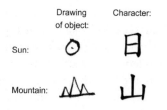

Figure 6 Some Chinese characters are pictographic – they developed originally from stylised drawings of the items they represent

is entirely pictographic – i.e. that it is a language in which its words or concepts are represented by single, complex characters. Some of its characters *do* represent entire words, and the shape of the character gives a clue to the word's meaning. For example, the characters for sun and mountain are shown in figure 6. Such characters are few, however.

The vast majority of Chinese characters include a semantic element, which provides information about the meaning of the character, and a phonetic element, which provides information about its pronunciation. For example, see the character for *mother* in figure 7.

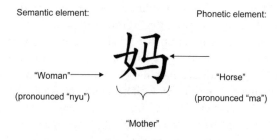

Figure 7 A Chinese character with phonetic and semantic elements

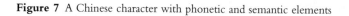

This is composed of the symbol for *woman*, which provides the meaning, and the symbol for *horse*, which provides a clue to the word's pronunciation but no information about meaning. However, the phonetic information is for the most part ambiguous. While the sounds that represent *horse* and *mother* in Chinese are both 'ma', they are pronounced in subtly different ways – 'ma' meaning mother is pronounced with a constant high pitch, while 'ma' meaning horse is pronounced with a low pitch that falls and then rises again. Confusingly, 'ma' can be pronounced in five ways, each having its own meaning. For this reason Chinese is considered to be a deep language.

The Japanese writing system has two forms – kanji and kana. Kanji is a pictographic script that was imported from China, and each kanji character can be pronounced in two ways. One way represents the original Chinese word form, the other the Japanese word form. Which of these is correct in any particular sentence is dictated by the context.

Kanji characters usually represent nouns (e.g. horse), and verb and adjective stems. For example, the kanji character that represents the verb 'to see' cannot be changed to represent the past tense ('saw'), the future tense ('will see'), or the negative ('do not see'). Similarly, the character that represents the adjective 'happy' cannot be changed into the comparative form ('happier') or the adverb ('happily'). These modifications are indicated by the presence of a kana character that follows the stem.

Kana is a phonetic script that reliably represents syllables in the spoken language. As you have just seen, it provides verb endings (e.g. to indicate past tense) and is also used to write foreign names and words for which there is no kanji character. While kanji characters provide no clue to their pronunciation, so are considered to be orthographically deep, kana characters have a perfect correspondence between their written form and their pronunciation, so they are considered to be orthographically shallow.

Although learning to read Chinese requires less obvious phonological processing than that involved in learning to read alphabetic languages, some phonological skills are still necessary. The finding that Chinese dyslexic readers experience similar phonological difficulties to dyslexic readers of alphabetic languages – including slower object naming, less accurate detection and production of rhymes, less accurate deletion of phonemes from spoken words, and less accurate repetition of non-words than other children of the same age – is, therefore, unsurprising. These poor phonological skills prevent dyslexic Chinese readers from benefiting from the phonological information provided by the phonetic elements of the printed characters.

As you saw in chapter 4, dyslexic readers tend to have difficulty analysing not only the sounds of words (phonology) but also the written forms of words (orthography). Given the complexity of Chinese written characters, dyslexic readers' orthographic difficulties are also likely to hinder their reading. This was explored in a large-scale study of dyslexic children in Hong Kong, which found that relative to unimpaired readers of the same age:

- 29% were significantly less able to detect onsets and rimes within words, and to repeat words and non-words accurately (i.e. they showed phonological difficulties).
- 42% showed significantly poorer knowledge of the structure of written characters (i.e. they showed orthographic difficulties).
- 27% showed poorer visual perception and visual memory (i.e. they showed visual perceptual difficulties).
- 57% were slower at naming written digits (i.e. they showed rapid naming difficulties).

As this particular study failed to test younger children of the same reading age it is difficult to know whether these deficits are a cause or a consequence of the dyslexic children's reading difficulties. It is possible that these children's poorer knowledge of the structure of written characters might result from them spending less time reading than unimpaired readers of the same age. Results from studies such as this one, however, suggest that Chinese children with dyslexia have fundamental impairments in processing the sounds and visual forms of the language just as dyslexic readers of alphabetic languages do.

A rather different picture emerges from studies of Japanese dyslexic readers. One interesting case study was reported by Taeko Wydell and Brian Butterworth of Brunel University and University College London. They described a sixteen-year-old boy – referred to as AS – who was introduced in the vignette at the start of this chapter. AS was born in Japan to an Australian father (who worked as a journalist and writer) and an English mother (who worked as an English teacher), and he grew up in Japan to be completely bilingual in English and Japanese. He was amongst the top 10% of readers of his age in Japanese, reading at a graduate level, but in English he was very dyslexic, displaying particular difficulty with reading, spelling, and phonological processing. Clearly, this boy's phonological difficulties existed whichever language he was reading, yet they only manifested themselves when he read a language (in this case English) that depends on complex and irregular spelling–sound translation. The regularity and consistency of Japanese presents no such difficulties.

To explain this dissociation, Wydell and Butterworth suggested that languages could be classified along two dimensions, representing (1) the transparency of the language – from transparent (shallow) to opaque (deep) languages; and (2) the granularity of the language – from fine (where words are read by breaking them down into letters that represent individual sounds) to coarse (where words are read as whole units). These dimensions are illustrated in figure 8, with transparency on the x axis and granularity on the y axis.

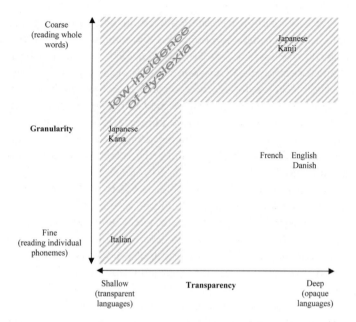

Figure 8 The incidence of dyslexia in languages that differ in transparency and granularity

The incidence of dyslexia will be low in: (1) any transparent language whether its granularity is fine (such as Italian), coarse, or anywhere in between (such as Japanese kana); and (2) any language with a coarse granularity whether the degree of transparency is high (e.g. Japanese kanji) or low. These combinations of transparency and granularity are illustrated by the hatched sections of figure 8.

By contrast, the incidence of dyslexia will be relatively high in opaque languages, particularly those which include fine to moderate grain sizes. This combination is illustrated by the non-hatched section of figure 8.

Because of its particular combination of transparency and granularity, Japanese is considered by some to be a perfect language for dyslexic readers to learn. This notion has been adopted enthusiastically by some schools in the UK which have selected Japanese to be their second language of choice, in preference to more traditionally taught European languages such as French, German, or Spanish. This move has been hailed a success, with many dyslexic pupils achieving a level of success with their foreign language studies that their predecessors had failed to reach.

So, to return to the question at the start of this chapter, is dyslexia universal? Dyslexia is found in speakers of many different languages both regular and irregular, alphabetic and non-alphabetic. Most dyslexic readers have difficulty processing the sounds of language. This manifests itself as poor verbal memory, slow naming of objects, and mispronunciation of multi-syllabic words. However, dyslexic readers of regular and irregular languages differ in the effects that these phonological difficulties have on their reading ability. Dyslexic readers of irregular languages read and spell slowly and inaccurately, while dyslexic readers of regular languages read and spell slowly but accurately. So it seems that dyslexia *is* universal although its signs and symptoms vary across languages.

In chapter 6 we'll consider the brain basis of normal and impaired reading development including a look at evidence for a universal neuro-anatomical basis of dyslexia.

6

Language on the brain

I think dyslexia should be described as ... er ... the physical manifestations are bad, basically are bad wiring of parts of the brain ... and it's a good way of explaining to someone who doesn't know, to describe dyslexia as a bad, or a badly wired part of the brain ... they find it easier to understand.

Chuck, a dyslexic reader (in *Dyslexia, the Self and Higher Education* by David Pollak, p. 165)

Reading and writing are artificial skills, evolutionary latecomers, appearing for the first time around 4000 BC in Sumeria (modern-day Iraq and Iran). This contrasts with speech, which first developed approximately 200–300,000 years ago. As reading and writing are such artificial and complex skills it is likely that the brain systems that support them are associated with pre-existing skills, such as the processing of speech, the production of gestures, visual processing, and verbal memory. These processes must interact in some remarkable way so that we can read and understand letters, words, and sentences, from the simplest *Janet and John* story to *Finnegan's Wake*.

We saw in chapter 1 that definitions of dyslexia generally include a statement that the disorder has a neurobiological or genetic origin. In this chapter we will look at evidence for the involvement of specific brain regions in language and reading-related processes.

Three pounds of cold porridge: a brief review of the brain

The brain is made up of two symmetrical-looking halves, or hemispheres. These two halves are independent but joined by a band of nerve fibres (the corpus callosum) which allows them to communicate with each other. The brain is made up of approximately 100 billion nerve cells (neurons) tightly packed within the confines of the skull. Because of this need to fit such a large amount of tissue into such a small space, the brain folds in on itself as it grows resulting in the pattern of bumps (gyri) and grooves (sulci) that you can see on the surface. If our brain tissue was unfolded and laid out flat it would cover an area of around 2,400 cm^2, or roughly the surface area of a twenty-seven-inch TV screen.

If you were to slice the brain in half horizontally from ear to ear the inner parts would look white in colour, hence it sometimes being referred to as white matter. The outside of the brain is slightly grey, so it is sometimes referred to as grey matter. Because of this grey and lumpy covering, the English mathematician Alan Turing described the brain as having the appearance of a bowl of cold porridge.

Unappealing breakfast fare aside, the outer surface of the brain is divided into four regions or lobes:

- The frontal lobe is associated with personality, forward planning, working memory, movement, and the inhibition of inappropriate behaviours.
- The parietal lobe is associated with visuospatial and sensory processing.
- The occipital lobe is associated with the processing of visual information.
- The temporal lobe is associated with the processing of language, memory, and sounds.

You can see the location of the lobes in figure 9.

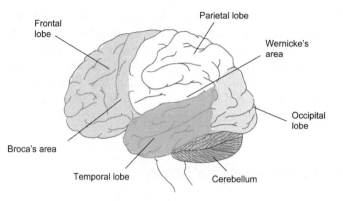

Figure 9 The lobes of the brain

Language areas in the brain

The study of the brain's language areas dates back to the mid-nineteenth century. The neurologists Pierre Paul Broca and Marc Dax observed that patients with brain damage to the front part of the left hemisphere lost the ability to produce fluent speech. The most famous of Broca's patients was a fifty-year-old man called Leborgne, known in the scientific literature as 'Tan' as this was the only sound he was able to produce without effort. Although otherwise healthy and intelligent, Tan seemed to understand the speech of others but lost the ability to speak articulately at the age of thirty years. Thereafter he went into a gradual physical decline, losing the use of his right arm, right leg, and the left side of his face. Following his death in 1861 he was found to have a cavity on the left side of his brain caused by a syphilitic lesion approximately the size of a chicken's egg. This lesion was located in the frontal lobe, just in front of the motor cortex. This part of the brain is now named Broca's area (shown in Figure 9).

A short time after this, Carl Wernicke studied a patient who had suffered a stroke after which he could produce speech but not understand it. Wernicke observed that his patient's stroke had caused damage to a region of his brain, again on the left side, but this time slightly further back than Broca's area, in the parietal/temporal region (shown in figure 9). This region is now named Wernicke's area.

Reading and the brain

The processes involved in reading and writing are not associated with any single part of the brain, but with many areas spread across the four lobes. These areas are associated with visual and auditory processing, language, memory, and movement.

The first stage of reading involves analysing the form of the written word. Light from the page enters the eyes and is converted into electrical signals; these signals are transmitted to the optic disk at the back of the eye. From the optic disk, visual information is sent via the optic nerve to a structure deep inside the brain, called the thalamus. The thalamus is a 'relay station' that receives sensory information – visual information from the eyes, auditory information from the ears, gustatory information from the taste buds, and somatic information from the skin – and passes it on to the part of the brain specialised to analyse it; so visual information is sent to the visual cortex, auditory information to the auditory cortex, and so on.

The visual cortex analyses the visual features of the letters on the page – their location, thickness, orientation, shape, and colour – although it does not recognise them as letters at this stage. This occurs when the information is sent to the angular gyrus, a region of the brain located at the junction of the occipital, temporal, and parietal cortices (see figure 10). As you saw in

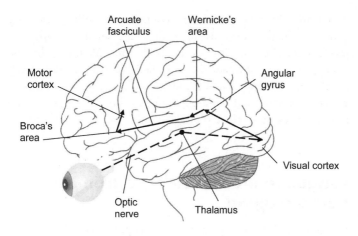

Figure 10 The reading pathway in the brain

chapter 1, the angular gyrus is where visual and auditory information is combined – where information from printed text is converted into its spoken form. So as we read, even silently to ourselves, we produce the sounds of the words and our brains analyse these sounds just as if we were listening to someone else speaking. Unsurprisingly, damage to the angular gyrus causes difficulties with reading and writing.

From the angular gyrus the sound of the spoken word is passed on to Wernicke's area where it is recognised and given meaning, and we understand what we have read. If we are to pronounce the word, the information is passed on again to Broca's area which contains memories of the muscle movements that we need to make to pronounce words. If we are to read the word silently then the memories stored in Broca's area enable us to 'say' the word, sub-vocally, to ourselves. If we are to read the word aloud, however, then information is passed on once again, to the motor cortex which controls the muscles of the lips, jaws, and tongue, and we speak.

Clearly, this is an over-simplified description of how the very complex brain allows us to read. This serial, step-by-step processing of information is not entirely true. We know that the brain processes information 'in parallel'. This means that many brain regions are activated simultaneously as the brain analyses visual, auditory, and semantic information to enable skilled readers to read quickly and efficiently.

Language areas: evidence from neuroimaging

In figure 11 you can see that the brain appears to be divided, top and bottom, by a line called the Sylvian fissure. The areas important for the production and comprehension of language lie around this fissure so they are sometimes referred to as peri-Sylvian regions. There are three main peri-Sylvian areas that are important for reading. These are:

1. The anterior language area ('anterior' referring to the front of the brain), including Broca's area. This area, and surrounding brain areas, play a role in the processing of syntax – making sense of the 'rules' of the language. For example, Broca's area is active when we try to make sense of ungrammatical sentences such as 'John drove home Sally in his new brand sports car' or grammatically complex sentences such as 'The shy young boy in the red jumper was bitten by the big black dog with the brown collar'.

2. The upper posterior language area ('posterior' referring to the back of the brain), lying between the temporal lobe and the parietal lobe. This includes Wernicke's area. This temporal-parietal region is more active when a person reads low

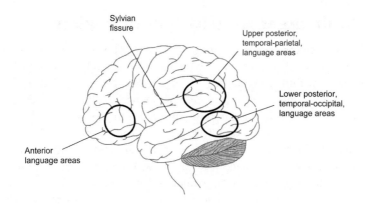

Figure 11 The three main language areas of the brain

frequency (uncommon) words and non-words than when he/she reads familiar, real words.

3. The lower posterior language area lies between the temporal lobe and the occipital lobe. It is active during skilled, automatic word recognition, Braille reading, and the naming of pictures, letters, and colours. This area is more active when skilled readers read familiar words than non-words, and when they read pronounceable non-words (e.g. *trolp*) than unpronounceable non-words (e.g. *xrilc*).

Anterior and posterior language areas become active during reading although precisely which regions are active depends on many factors. For example:

- whether the individual is a skilled reader or a novice reader;
- whether they are reading out loud or silently;
- whether they are reading real words or non-words;
- whether they are a dyslexic or non-dyslexic reader;
- the language that they are reading.

Brain areas used by novice readers

Young children who are just learning to read need to analyse all printed words that they are trying to understand. The individual letters within a word (e.g. *c*, *a*, *t*) must be recognised and converted into their corresponding sounds ('kuh', 'ah', 'tuh'), before being combined into the spoken word 'cat' that the child can then understand as referring to a small, furry animal that meows. This novice reading is linked with brain activity in the upper posterior language area, including Wernicke's area, and in the anterior language area, including Broca's area.

As you have seen, these brain regions are associated with analysing, articulating, and remembering sounds. They are active during the reading of low frequency, unfamiliar words, and non-words. Of course, to young children who are just learning to read, most words are unfamiliar and of low frequency, so activity in these regions is associated with slow, letter-by-letter reading.

Brain areas used by skilled readers

As reading skills develop children become increasingly familiar with written words and learn to recognise them by sight. This skilled reading is associated with brain activity in the posterior temporal-occipital language area and also, to a lesser extent, in part of Broca's area.

More activity is seen in the posterior language area when skilled readers read familiar words compared with when they read unfamiliar non-words. This is also the case when they read pronounceable non-words compared with when they read unpronounceable non-words. This region is responsible, therefore, for the skilled, automatic recognition of words.

As reading skill increases so does the speed with which our

brains respond when we look at a word. Within 100–150 milliseconds of seeing a word (that is, within 100–150 thousandths of a second) the visual cortex becomes active. Within 200 milliseconds activity is seen in the temporal-occipital brain region as the word is identified. Within 200–600 milliseconds activity occurs in Broca's area as we say the word sub-vocally to ourselves, and around 400 milliseconds (400 thousandths of a second) after seeing a familiar word activity occurs in Wernicke's area and we understand the word's meaning.

Dyslexic brains and non-dyslexic brains: do they look different?

As noted earlier, on casual inspection the two halves of the brain appear to be approximately symmetrical. Closer inspection though reveals some interesting differences. Brain imaging studies and post-mortem examinations have highlighted regions in the left hemisphere that are larger (and sulci that are longer) than corresponding regions in the right hemisphere. These regions in the frontal, temporal, and parietal lobes of the brain are known to be involved in auditory processing and in the production and comprehension of language. The ability to produce and comprehend language has been associated with a significant development in the size of these regions in the left hemisphere and with reduction in size of the same regions in the right hemisphere. One region in particular, called the planum temporale, can be up to five times larger in the left hemisphere than in the right. Some researchers have shown that the larger these left hemisphere regions are relative to those in the right hemisphere, the better the individual's reading and phonological processing skills.

Regions of the temporal lobe, including the planum temporale, are found to be symmetrical in the majority (about 70%) of dyslexic brains. Parts of the parietal and occipital lobes are also larger in the right than left hemisphere of dyslexic brains. These abnormal patterns of symmetry/asymmetry have been associated with poorer language skills including poor phonological processing. What is surprising, however, is that these structural abnormalities in dyslexic brains are not the result of smaller than expected regions in the left hemisphere, but of larger than expected regions in the right hemisphere. This may be the result of insufficient 'pruning' of cells in the right hemisphere. As the brain matures cells that are ineffective or unused normally die off spontaneously. This is a normal developmental process that allows the remaining cells to form a more efficient network. It would appear that the lack of pruning in dyslexic brains results in an abnormal brain structure. As brain regions involved in the processing of language are usually larger in the left hemisphere than in the right then symmetry, or reversed asymmetry, of these regions may disturb normal language development and increase the risk of developmental language disorders.

A team of neuroscientists at Harvard Medical School, led by Al Galaburda, examined eight brains of dyslexic readers post-mortem to identify possible structural differences between these brains and brains taken from non-dyslexic readers. The team observed microscopic irregularities called ectopias in the structure of the dyslexic readers' brain tissue. These ectopias, described as 'disorganised islands of cortex' or 'brain warts', usually develop in the first six months of gestation. In a typically developing brain, after cells are formed they move to their final location and form connections with neighbouring cells; this process is controlled by our genes. However, sometimes this process goes wrong. When it does cells move to the wrong location within the brain, they become malformed and form abnormal connections with other cells.

Although ectopias are not unknown in the brains of non-dyslexic readers they are rare and generally occur in the right temporal lobe. In dyslexic brains they have mostly been seen in the language regions of the left hemisphere around the junction of the temporal and parietal lobes, but especially the planum temporale. These ectopias seem to have two effects on the dyslexic brain:

1. They remove the leftward asymmetry which is typically seen in the language areas. None of the dyslexic brains studied by Galaburda and colleagues showed leftward asymmetry of the planum temporale.
2. They alter the connections between and within the language areas. Anything which disturbs the normal structure and function of the brain's language areas is likely to cause difficulties with reading, writing, spelling, and the processing of language, as seen in dyslexia.

Post-mortem examination of dyslexic brains has also shown clusters of cells in the thalamus that are smaller than expected and abnormal in structure. As we have seen, the thalamus receives rapid visual and auditory information from the eyes and ears and sends this on to other regions of the brain which are responsible for processing it. Irregularities in the size and structure of cells in the thalamus are likely to impair the speed and efficiency of processing of rapid visual and auditory information. This might explain some of the phonological and visual processing difficulties of dyslexia (returned to later in the chapter).

Dyslexia and testosterone

One theory of dyslexia suggests that abnormal brain development results from hormonal influences in the pre-natal period. This theory assumes a *standard* pattern of brain dominance in the majority of people, with the left side of the brain controlling language and also handedness. As the right hand is controlled by the left hemisphere of the brain, and the left hand by the right hemisphere, most people will be right-handed.

According to this hypothesis an excess of foetal testosterone (the male sex hormone) retards the development of the left side of the brain allowing the right side to develop to a greater degree. This enhancement of the right side of the brain is thought to increase the probability of developmental disorders including dyslexia, and also left-handedness. (The link between handedness and dyslexia will be re-visited in the next chapter.) However, the suggestion that high levels of testosterone impair development of the left hemisphere in foetuses has been challenged.

It is not possible to measure concentrations of pre-natal testosterone to see the effects that changing levels have on subsequent development of the foetus. To circumvent this problem, some researchers have pointed to the relative length of individuals' second and fourth fingers (counting the thumb as the first finger) as an indirect indication of pre-natal testosterone. Exposure to high levels of pre-natal testosterone has been linked with a shorter second than fourth finger while exposure to low levels of pre-natal testosterone has been linked with second and fourth fingers that are similar in length.

Studies comparing the relative finger length of dyslexic and non-dyslexic readers, however, have failed to find significant differences between these two groups. This may be because the length of the fingers – and the development of the skeleton in general – is determined within the first few weeks of gestation, while most of the brain's growth occurs much later. For example, changes in the structure of the brain associated with dyslexia occur around the sixth month of gestation. It might well be that fluctuations in testosterone concentration throughout the pregnancy have different effects at different stages of development, and relative finger length may reveal very little about the possible link between pre-natal testosterone and dyslexia.

Furthermore, contrary to expectations people with adrenogenital syndrome – a rare congenital disorder characterised by abnormally high levels of pre-natal testosterone – show normal brain development, good verbal intelligence, and right-handedness.

Therefore, if abnormally high levels of pre-natal testosterone do not result in dyslexia, and people with dyslexia cannot be shown to have higher than expected levels of testosterone, then we must be extremely sceptical about the role that pre-natal testosterone may play in dyslexia.

Do dyslexic brains function differently?

Unsurprisingly, the answer to this question is yes. Dyslexic readers and skilled readers show differences in activity in various brain areas including the visual system and in all three of the peri-Sylvian language regions.

Dyslexia and the visual pathway

Historically, dyslexia was considered to be a visual disorder and research has focused on the visual system, especially the role of the thalamus, in the reading problems of dyslexia. The thalamus contains two main types of cell:

1. magnocells, or 'large cells' which detect orientation, movement, direction, and depth, and direct eye movements to enable individuals to maintain steady fixation of the eyes on a visual target; and

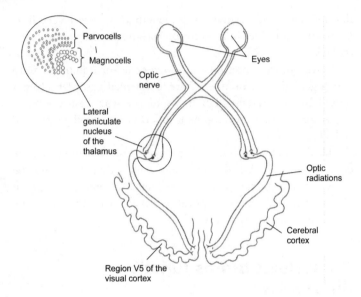

Figure 12 The visual system

2. parvocells, or 'small cells' which detect colour and fine detail (see figure 12).

Post-mortem evidence has shown that in some dyslexic readers' brains magnocells are around 30% smaller than those in the brains of non-dyslexic readers. These cells are also more *disorganised* in their arrangement in dyslexic brains. In non-dyslexic brains the magnocells and parvocells are arranged in discrete layers whereas in dyslexic brains the two types of cells are mixed together. Although it is unclear precisely how the abnormal size and arrangement of magnocells affects their function, they may disrupt the fast and efficient transmission of information through the visual system.

Information from the magnocells is sent for analysis to part of the visual cortex located within the temporal lobe. This region, called region V5, is shown in figure 12. If dyslexic readers' magnocells are functioning abnormally, this should be reflected in lack of activity in area V5. In a brain imaging study by Guinevere Eden, dyslexic and non-dyslexic men were asked to look at stationary dots and moving dots on a computer screen while their brain activity was measured. While the non-dyslexic readers showed the expected pattern of increased activity in V5 in the left and right sides of the brain in response to the moving dots, none of the dyslexic readers did. No differences were found in the dyslexic and non-dyslexic readers' brain activity when viewing stationary dots.

Although activity *can* be seen in region V5 in dyslexic readers' brains, this activity may be less when compared with non-dyslexic readers. Furthermore, it has been shown that the greater the activity in V5, the greater the reading speed and proficiency in both dyslexic and non-dyslexic readers.

The precise role that region V5 plays in dyslexia is currently unclear, but it is possible that inactivity in this region in dyslexic brains is linked to the underlying visual system abnormalities described in chapter 4. As we saw, the abnormal size and arrangement of magnocells in the visual system disrupts the fast and efficient transmission of visual information. This disruption may manifest itself as inactivity in region V5 at the 'other end' of the system.

Dyslexia and the language areas: evidence from neuroimaging

There have been relatively few brain imaging studies of dyslexia, but evidence so far indicates that dyslexic and non-dyslexic readers activate the brain's anterior and posterior language areas in a different way when they read.

In one study of eight- to thirteen-year-old dyslexic and non-dyslexic boys, the children listened to pairs of words while their brain activity was measured. The word pairs were either rhyming words (e.g. *fly/eye*), non-rhyming words (e.g. *fly/church*), a non-word plus a rhyming real word (e.g. *treel/meal*), or a non-word plus a non-rhyming real word (e.g. *treel/crow*). The boys were asked whether the words rhymed. Activity was almost five times greater in and around Broca's area in the dyslexic boys' brains compared with the non-dyslexic boys'. It is possible that this hyper-activation seen in the anterior language areas may reflect dyslexic readers' sounding-out of words sub-vocally to support their poor phonological skills and their poor visual identification of printed text when reading.

Studies with dyslexic adults have shown similar over-activation in anterior language regions alongside under-activation, or lack of activation, in posterior language regions. One region that is particularly affected is the angular gyrus at the junction of the occipital, temporal, and parietal cortices. This region converts printed text into its spoken representation. The absence of activity in this region in dyslexic readers has led some researchers to identify the angular gyrus as a key region in dyslexia. If this region fails to work in concert with the other language areas, then information will not be passed effectively from the posterior to the anterior language areas and the individual will experience reading and writing problems.

Others have found consistent under-activation, or lack of activation, in the lower posterior language area when dyslexic readers read strings of letters silently, look at printed concrete and abstract words, read non-words, and read real words out loud. Dyslexic readers even show less activity here than do non-dyslexic readers during picture naming when no text is involved.

This over-activation in anterior language regions associated with letter-by-letter reading, and under-activation in posterior regions associated with automatic word recognition, seems to reflect an effortful decoding strategy employed by dyslexic readers. This strategy may help them to compensate to some extent for their difficulties in accessing whole words in their mental lexicon.

A study of English, Italian, and French dyslexic readers has found a consistent lack of activity in the left temporal-occipital cortex and other language areas during explicit and implicit reading, as shown in figure 13. Remember from chapter 5 that these three languages differ in the regularity of their spelling-sound relationships – English is a highly irregular language, Italian is a highly regular language, French lies somewhere between the two. This suggests that dyslexia may have a common origin in English, Italian, and French speakers irrespective of the language in which they speak and read.

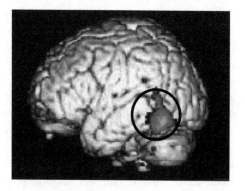

Figure 13 English, Italian, and French dyslexic readers showed consistent lack of activity in the temporal-occipital cortex when reading

Dyslexia and disconnection

As well as showing differences in the activity of anterior and posterior language areas during reading, it is possible that dyslexic brains are also 'wired' together differently such that the language regions are *functionally disconnected*. It is important to note that functional disconnection is not the same as anatomical, physical disconnection. Two brain areas may be physically connected but functionally disconnected. In this case when one area becomes active during reading, naming, or the performance of some other task, the other does not.

This suggestion of functional disconnection in dyslexia was first made by the team of English and Italian researchers, headed by Uta Frith and Eraldo Paulesu, whose cross-cultural study was described in chapter 5. They asked dyslexic and non-dyslexic university students to perform a visual rhyme judgement task (e.g. do the letters *d* and *p* rhyme?) and a visual short-term memory task (e.g. was the letter *t* present in a string of letters that you just saw?). The researchers found that the non-dyslexic readers showed activity in anterior and posterior language areas, and connecting areas in between, during both tasks. The dyslexic readers, however, showed activity only in posterior language areas during the short-term memory task, and only in anterior language areas during the rhyme judgement task. They showed no activity in the connecting brain regions.

Others have found evidence of disconnection between the language areas in dyslexic brains, for example, between the angular gyrus and the temporal-occipital cortex, and between the angular gyrus and Wernicke's area.

This lack of proper functional connection between language areas may result in inefficient communication between these areas, and this is likely to impede the development of automatic language processing skills in dyslexic readers' brains.

The finding that dyslexic brains function differently to non-dyslexic brains is summed up in the following matter-of-fact way by Eileen Simpson:

> It did not surprise me to learn that the seat of [dyslexia] is in the brain. In my own case I had localized it there at the age of nine. (I had even felt ... a *brain*ache, which is quite different from a headache.) The jamming, blocking, and confusion I suffered from I had likened to a mechanical breakdown – an out-of-order switchboard, two typewriter keys locking so that neither prints.

> *Reversals. A Personal Account of Victory over Dyslexia*, p. 205

The question of real practical interest, of course, is whether these observed differences – this 'mechanical breakdown' – can be corrected through therapy or training to improve dyslexic readers' ability to read and write.

Can intervention change the way that dyslexic brains work?

A number of interesting studies in the last few years has shown that it is possible to change the brain regions that dyslexic readers use when they read. In these studies individuals receive intensive instruction in reading-related skills – including word decoding, reading comprehension, and phonological processing – for several hours a day over the course of a few months.

In some of these studies dyslexic children participated in an eight-week, commercially available, phonological training programme for up to three hours a day, five days a week. This training involved children playing computer games designed to teach phonological skills through the use of artificially slowed and amplified computer-generated speech. The speed of the speech was increased gradually over the training period. The games in the training program included:

1. Phonic match. Children are shown grids of brightly-coloured squares. When each square is clicked with the computer mouse, the computer speaks a simple word (e.g. *but, buck, dug, tug*). The child is asked to identify the pairs of squares within the grid that are associated with the same word.

2. Phonic word. The game shows pairs of objects that differ in their first sound, middle sound, or last sound. For example, the pictures show a baseball *base* and a *face*, and the child is asked to point to the base, or the pictures show a *fan* and a *fang* and the child is asked to point to the fang.

3. Phoneme identification. An animated character speaks a simple target sound (e.g. 'ba'). Two other characters then speak – one the target sound, the other a similar, distracter sound (e.g. 'ga'). The child is asked to point to the character that produced the target sound.

Brain activity in children who participated in these studies changed significantly over time. Before training the children showed large areas of right hemisphere activity but little activity in the left hemisphere's language areas during the completion of a phonological processing task. In this task, children were asked to decide whether pairs of visually presented letters rhymed (e.g. *T* and *G* rhyme, but *L* and *R* do not). After the eight weeks these children's brains showed significantly more activity in the left hemisphere, particularly in the anterior language region and the posterior, temporal-parietal region. This pattern of activity was almost equivalent to that of non-dyslexic readers, so the researchers described the training as having 'normalized' the dyslexic children's brain activity. Furthermore, the dyslexic readers' word and non-word reading, and reading comprehension, had also improved following the training. Children who showed the greatest activation in the left hemisphere temporal-parietal region also showed the greatest improvement in non-word reading ability and phonological processing following training.

As well as increases in left hemisphere activity, significant increases were also seen in the dyslexic readers' brains in various right hemisphere regions – across the frontal, temporal, and parietal lobes – after training. The researchers suggest that these changes reflected 'compensating effects of remediation', i.e. brain regions that were not normally responsible for language production and comprehension took on this role after a period of training. This compensation is commonly seen in children and adults following brain damage, where non-damaged brain regions take over the function of damaged regions.

It is also possible that this right hemisphere activity reflects differences in the wiring of dyslexic and non-dyslexic brains. Given that connections between corresponding anterior and posterior regions in the right hemisphere in dyslexic readers are strong, it is possible that the intensive phonological training received by the dyslexic children enhanced these already strong right hemisphere connections.

Dyslexia and the cerebellum

There may be one other region of the brain which has an important role to play in dyslexia: the cerebellum. This lies at the base of the brain (shown in figure 9), and there seem to be differences in the structure of the cerebellum in dyslexic and non-dyslexic readers. While the cerebella of non-dyslexic brains are typically asymmetrical, larger on the right side than on the left, those of dyslexic brains are typically more symmetrical. Furthermore, in dyslexic readers the more symmetrical the cerebellum the poorer their ability to read non-words.

However, it would be wrong to assume that symmetry of the cerebellum in some way causes the problems of dyslexia, or that cerebellar symmetry and dyslexia are caused by some other common factor. We know that the development of the brain is shaped by our experiences, and research has shown that the side of the cerebellum that controls the writing hand is smaller in dyslexic adults than in unimpaired readers. This difference in size may reflect nothing more than that dyslexic readers are less likely than non-dyslexic readers to spend time writing because it is a task that they find frustrating and difficult. Consequently, the cerebellum would not show the same level of development in dyslexic readers as in individuals with a history of well-practised writing.

The cerebellum has a number of functions. Traditionally its role was thought to be largely limited to the control of movement, posture, and balance. It constantly receives sensory information about the location of our bodies in space and if necessary, sends signals to the muscles to adjust our posture and balance as we move around. It is also involved in the automatisation of motor skills. As a new skill is mastered, the amount of conscious attention that we need to pay to it decreases and the skill becomes automatic.

More recently a role has been suggested for the cerebellum in the processing of spoken language and in reading. Regions of the cerebellum become consistently active when non-dyslexic readers compare pairs of written words to see if they rhyme (e.g. *rice* and *mice*), and when they compare pairs of words to see if they belong to the same semantic category (e.g. *man* and *boy*). Patients with cerebellar damage display poor verbal fluency and they have difficulty understanding grammar in spoken language. Impaired functioning of the cerebellum is also being increasingly identified as a key factor in dyslexia.

Many dyslexic children tend to be clumsy and uncoordinated, experiencing difficulty with actions such as catching a

ball, tying their shoelaces, or riding a bicycle. They have difficulty achieving fluency in new skills, needing to expend a great
deal of effort to be able to perform tasks or actions automatically.
And of course they have difficulty with reading and with spoken
language production and comprehension. All of these difficulties
might be explained by poor functioning of the cerebellum.

There seems to be less cerebellar activity in the brains of
dyslexic readers than in the brains of non-dyslexic readers when
they read and when they perform simple motor tasks, such as
tapping out rhythms with their fingers. Considering how important the cerebellum is in the control of movement, you may be
unsurprised by the latter finding, but what about the former?
Why should dyslexic readers show less activity in the cerebellum
than non-dyslexic readers when they read? As we have seen,
reading is a complicated activity that involves many component
skills; these must be practised and developed until they become
over-learned and automatic just like any other skilled motor
behaviour. So, the relative lack of automaticity in the reading of
dyslexic children and adults may explain the relative lack of
cerebellar activation.

Clearly, brain development is an extremely complex process
that is influenced by environmental factors such as pre-natal
exposure to toxins and malnutrition, and experience, including
sensory and linguistic stimulation during infancy and childhood.
The other major influence on an individual's brain development
is their genetic makeup. Chapter 7 will consider the role of
genes in dyslexia.

7

A problem of faulty genes?

My mother was the genetic link to my dyslexia. What I had learned … was that my disability was not unique. My mother had had it … Was my grandmother also dyslexic? I had no evidence that she was. From whom my mother's inheritance came, I don't know. Had I had children there is a good chance that one of them would have inherited the disability from me.

Reversals. A Personal Account of Victory over Dyslexia
by Eileen Simpson, p. 98.

Dyslexia seems to run in families. Most people with dyslexia can identify a family member – a brother, father, aunt – who is also dyslexic, or who experienced reading difficulties. Around 33–43% of dyslexic readers will have a history of dyslexia in their family. If an adult with dyslexia has a child there is a 40–60% probability that the child will develop the disorder, although this figure may increase if other close family members are also affected.

Some of the earliest studies of dyslexia identified multiple cases within the same family. This style of research, in which all available family members are tested for a particular trait such as eye colour, handedness, or the presence of an illness or disorder, is still undertaken today. These studies reveal a lot about the way in which traits are passed from parents to children (i.e. about their heritability).

A particular type of study used to investigate the genetic basis of dyslexia involves twins. Research determines the extent to which identical and non-identical twins share particular traits. Identical twins grow from a single egg so they share 100% of their genes. Non-identical twins grow from two eggs so they share on average 50% of their genes, the same as any other two siblings. Knowing this we can make two predictions about the heritability of dyslexia:

1. If dyslexia is genetic, then if one identical twin develops it so will the other, i.e. the likelihood of both twins having dyslexia will be higher in identical twins than in non-identical twins.
2. If dyslexia is not genetic but is caused instead by some factor in the environment – e.g. poor teaching or lack of reading practice at home – then the likelihood of dyslexia in identical and non-identical twins will be the same, i.e. they will be equally affected by the school and home environments.

Twin studies have shown that if one identical twin is dyslexic, the other twin has a 68% likelihood of being dyslexic. If one non-identical twin is dyslexic, the other twin has a 38% likelihood of being dyslexic. These figures show that dyslexia does indeed have a strong genetic basis but it is not entirely genetically determined otherwise the figure for identical twins would be 100% and not 68%.

But what does this actually mean? Is there a gene that dyslexic readers inherit from their parents that *gives* them dyslexia? Not really. Reading is a 'cultural invention', a man-made skill, for which there can be no specific gene. However, our genes do control the growth of brain regions responsible for the perception and analysis of visual and verbal information, skills which are necessary for reading. As we saw in the previous chapter, successful reading depends on the development of a particular structure and function of the brain. Anything that causes this structure or function to develop atypically is likely to predispose the individual to have reading (and general language) difficulties. The most obvious factor that can influence the development of the brain is, of course, our genes.

The inheritance of particular combinations of genes may predispose someone to be a good reader or to be dyslexic, although the way this occurs is far from simple. As Professor Robert Plomin from London's Institute of Psychiatry points out:

> for complex things like talent … it's many genes, each having a small effect. Even at the extreme end of behaviour – say a child who can't read – you might find heredity accounting for 60% of the trait. But the relevant genes won't actually be very different from those of a child who can read normally.

We inherit twenty-three chromosomes from each of our parents. These join together to give us twenty-three pairs, or forty-six individual chromosomes, comprising 20–30,000 genes that provide the instructions for our development. The development of dyslexia has been linked with information stored on various chromosomes, including numbers 1, 2, 3, 6, 15, and 18 (see figure 14). Information on these chromosomes has been associated with variations in phonological processing, orthographic processing, rapid naming, verbal short-term memory, and reading and spelling ability.

One study tested thirty members of a Norwegian family, amongst whom eleven dyslexic readers were identified. Blood samples taken from these individuals enabled researchers to locate a gene – identified as gene DYX3 on chromosome 2 – that may underlie this family's reading difficulties. The role played by gene DYX3 in dyslexia has been confirmed by a larger study of ninety-six Canadian families – 877 individuals – each containing at least two children with dyslexia.

Another gene – identified as DCDC2 on chromosome 6 – was found by researchers who tested (genotyped) 153 families with dyslexic family members. This gene normally controls the structural development of the brain's language areas in the

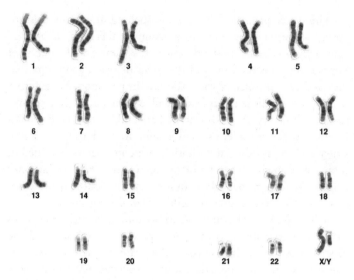

Figure 14 The twenty-three pairs of chromosomes that we inherit from our parents

embryo. Any genetic abnormality in DCDC2 is believed to disrupt the architecture of the language areas as dyslexic brains develop pre-natally. Professor Jeffrey Gruen, the lead researcher of the study claimed that:

> We now have strong statistical evidence that a large number of dyslexic cases – perhaps as many as 20% – are due to the DCDC2 gene.

However, while many dyslexic readers may have this faulty gene (although clearly, most may not), it has not yet been shown that all people with this faulty gene develop dyslexia. Much more research is still needed.

Other candidate genes for dyslexia include DYX1C1 on chromosome 15, KIAA0319 on chromosome 6, and ROBO1 on chromosome 3.

The development of reading and spelling impairments is not purely the result of our genes. Environmental factors, such as the language spoken by the individual, the nature and quality of their reading instruction, and the level of reading support that they receive, also play a role. We saw in previous chapters that an English child with dyslexia will experience much greater reading difficulty than will an Italian child with dyslexia. An English dyslexic reader who is taught to read using a highly structured, supportive, and multi-sensory approach (described in more detail in chapter 8) will fare much better than will another English dyslexic reader whose dyslexia is not identified and who, as a consequence, receives no additional reading support.

Much more work still needs to be done to identify the genes that could contribute to the development of dyslexia, and the precise effects that they have in the brains of dyslexic readers. The sooner the full genetic profile associated with dyslexia is known, the sooner children can be identified early in life as exhibiting this profile and be given the specialist educational help that they need to prevent them falling behind at school. This will particularly benefit children who are disadvantaged by speaking an orthographically deep language.

Handedness and dyslexia

Some research suggests that left-handedness and mixed-handedness – where individuals show no strong preference for either hand – is more common amongst dyslexic than non-dyslexic readers. The right hand is controlled largely by the left side of the brain and the left hand by the right side. So, if the growth of the left side of the brain is impeded – by testosterone, for example, as discussed in the previous chapter, or by genetic abnormality – while the right side continues to grow, this will hinder the development of the left hemisphere's language areas and increase the likelihood of mixed- or left-handedness.

There is some evidence to support this suggestion. Some researchers, for example, found that around 11% of dyslexic readers are left-handed compared with around 6% of non-dyslexic readers. Others have looked at the relationship from a different angle and found that language disorders (including dyslexia) occur in around 7–11% of left-handers compared with around 1% of right-handers.

Most research, however, finds no consistent link between dyslexia and handedness. A study of 407 dyslexic children and 604 non-dyslexic children found no statistically significant difference between the groups in the number of strong right-handers or strong left-handers. Furthermore, within the group of dyslexic children, those who were left-handed did not differ in the severity of their dyslexia from those who were right-handed. The inconsistency of the relationship between handed-ness and dyslexia is encapsulated in the following recollection by Eileen Simpson:

> As for that red herring, handedness, I was a clear-cut example
> of mixed dominance: left-handed, -eared, and -eyed at birth,
> right-handed by training. In periods when I had looked for a
> scapegoat to blame my failures on, I had blamed my first grade
> teacher for changing my writing hand. It was disconcerting to
> discover that my left-handed nephew, whose writing hand had
> also been changed, showed not a trace of dyslexia; whereas my
> niece's son who is dyslexic … is an unchanged left-hander.
>
> *Reversals. A Personal Account of Victory over Dyslexia*, p. 205

Also, the side of the brain which is dominant for language is not always the one that controls the dominant hand. Right-handed people do not always produce and comprehend language predominantly in the left side of their brains – although approx-imately 95% do – and left-handed people do not always produce and comprehend language in the right side of their brains – around 15% do. The vast majority produce and comprehend language in the left side of their brains just like the majority of right-handers.

So while the hypothesis is intuitively appealing, it is flawed. What we can conclude with certainty, however, is that whatever the relationship between handedness and dyslexia, most dyslexic readers are not left-handed and most left-handed people are not dyslexic.

Dyslexia and the immune system

We saw earlier that dyslexia has been linked with abnormality of a gene on chromosome 6 (amongst others). This gene – DCDC2 – normally controls the development of the brain's language areas but in dyslexia the structure of these areas is changed. Chromosome 6 has also been linked with the functioning of the immune system and with the presence of various immune disorders and allergies. Immune disorders such as rheumatoid arthritis, Crohn's disease, and ulcerative colitis cause a person's immune system to attack their own body. Allergies such as hay fever, eczema, and asthma cause an excessive reaction to a substance in the environment.

Some researchers have found an increase in immune disorders and allergies in dyslexic readers. Around 10% of dyslexic readers, but only around 1.5% of their non-dyslexic relatives, are thought to have an autoimmune disease. For allergies (particularly hay fever), the figures are around 30% and 12%. Conversely, people with immune diseases are reported to have a higher than expected number of relatives who are dyslexic. One study found that sons of women with lupus (a chronic disease in which the immune system attacks the major organs of the body) were almost four times as likely to have a learning disability, including dyslexia, than were sons of healthy women. No increased risk was found for daughters. Others have found no link between immune disorders and dyslexia although it is possible that only a sub-group of dyslexic readers (probably males) are at elevated risk of developing immune disorders and allergies.

If dyslexia is linked with immune disorders and allergies, then this may be caused by the presence of maternal auto-antibodies during the development of the embryo. Antibodies are proteins produced by the immune system that are designed to protect the individual against foreign organisms. Auto-antibodies attack the self instead of foreign organisms. In pregnant women 'the self' includes both the mother and the foetus. Mothers of dyslexic children have been found to produce twenty times the level of auto-antibodies produced by mothers of non-dyslexic children. The presence of auto-antibodies might cause the subtle structural abnormalities associated with dyslexia. It might also increase the likelihood of the child developing one or more immune disorders.

Alternatively, it is possible that the link between immune disorders and dyslexia may be caused by impaired functioning of the mother's immune system. This would expose the foetus to viruses which might bring about an inflammatory response in the foetus. Too great a response – too much inflammation – could affect the development of the foetus's brain structure. Support for this suggestion is provided by the finding that more dyslexic readers are born during spring and early summer than at any other time of year. These individuals, therefore, would have been exposed to a greater number of environmental toxins (which are more prevalent during the winter months) around the crucial sixth month of gestation.

This potential link between dyslexia and an abnormally functioning immune system brings us back to a possible role for essential fatty acids in dyslexia. Remember from chapter 4 that impaired functioning of cells in the eyes has been linked to a dietary deficiency of essential fatty acids. Research since the late 1990s has pointed out how important these fatty acids (such as omega-3) are for the normal development and function of the brain, and for effective functioning of the immune system. They do this by inhibiting the inflammatory response. Fatty acids cannot be produced by the body, they must come from dietary sources – from oily fish, such as mackerel, herring, or salmon, and from various seed oils; they are also present in breast milk. However, intake of these foods has generally decreased in the last few years, and many people are believed to be omega-3 deficient. It is these omega-3-deficient people who may benefit from increasing their dietary intake of essential fatty acids, or from taking fish oil supplements. A small number of studies has found that increasing the intake of omega-3 can improve reading and spelling in people who were previously omega-3 deficient. Much more research is still needed, however, to clarify the link between dyslexia, immune system functioning, and essential fatty acids.

Understanding the genetic and biological bases of dyslexia is important. As you have seen in this chapter, our knowledge of which genes are involved in dyslexia is increasing. So too is our understanding of how these genes change the structure and function of the dyslexic brain. Increasingly sophisticated brain scanning techniques allow us to explore similarities and differences between dyslexic and non-dyslexic brains. One day we may be able to diagnose dyslexia quickly and easily in children before they start to experience reading difficulties, before they start school, possibly even before they are born. However, that day is most likely a long way off. In the meantime we must continue to rely on paper-based and computer-based tests for the screening and assessment of dyslexia. These are described in chapter 8 along with strategies for managing dyslexia in daily life.

8

Assessing and managing dyslexia

> For a dyslexic who does not yet know they are dyslexic, life is like a big high wall you never think you will be able to climb or get over. The moment you understand there is something called dyslexia, and there are ways of getting around the problem, the whole world opens up.
>
> Sir Jackie Stewart (Formula One racing driver)

Unidentified, dyslexia can lead to children being labelled as lazy or just slow to develop. Parents who express concerns that their children might have dyslexia can all too often be dismissed by teachers with the assurance that 'children develop at different rates' or 'don't worry, all children learn to read in time'. As noted in chapter 1, some people in the UK have traditionally thought of dyslexia as a 'middle-class disease', an excuse made by middle-class parents to justify the slow reading progress being made by their children. However, as time progresses and the children continue to fail with their reading, it begins to have a wider effect on their schooling as reading difficulties affect their learning of all school subjects. In this situation some children may withdraw into themselves, become frustrated and disillusioned, and make excuses not to go to school. Their self-esteem and motivation plummet. Other children may become disruptive in the classroom, becoming the class clown to draw attention away from their reading difficulties. Such behaviour is exemplified by journalist Sophy Fisher who, commenting on her own school experience, wrote:

> I see children today doing everything I did to try to stop people
> seeing their failings – disrupting the class, lurking at the back,
> faking illness, losing homework. I even learnt the textbooks by
> heart, to hide the fact that I couldn't read them. Letters on a
> page appeared a meaningless jumble – with no more logic than
> alphabet spaghetti. I could never remember if the lines went
> from left-to-right, or right-to-left ... But in my small village
> school, I couldn't really hide the fact that I was the class idiot.

Many dyslexic children progress through school only with great
effort and high levels of anxiety. The difficulty of undiagnosed
dyslexia is summed up by Kid Chaos (real name Stephen Harris),
rock bassist and guitarist of, variously, *The Cult* and *Guns 'N'
Roses*:

> I'd spent my whole life at the bottom of the educational totem
> pole. It was painful. Every time I was in a classroom, it felt like
> a nightmare, and I thought everyone's learning experience was
> like that.

In an interview with *USA Today* in 2005 he told how his
dyslexia went undiagnosed in school causing him, at the age of
eleven, to abandon his plans to become a doctor. He turned
instead to music and at the age of eighteen achieved success
playing bass guitar in various rock bands. His rock career flour-
ished for the next seventeen years until, at the age of thirty-five,
he decided to pursue his original ambition of becoming a
doctor. On gaining a place in college he was finally diagnosed
with dyslexia and given the support that he needed to help him
to pursue his studies. He graduated from college and is currently
studying medicine at Columbia University in New York City.

The fortunate ones, or those with the highest levels of determination and support like Stephen, may go on to higher education. Around 40–50% of dyslexic readers are diagnosed at college
or university. The less fortunate ones, or those with the lowest

levels of determination and support, may truant from school, gain no qualifications, become unable to find employment, and turn to crime. Around 40% of prisoners in the UK are thought to be dyslexic. Thankfully, it doesn't have to be this way.

Research is now teaching us more about the strengths and difficulties of dyslexic readers, and this knowledge is being used to develop more detailed screening and assessment procedures that can identify dyslexia early on. In many countries around the world schools are now legally responsible for the identification and support of pupils with special educational needs. This support includes providing specialist teachers, using literacy teaching methods which benefit dyslexic and non-dyslexic pupils alike, and making special exam/assessment arrangements for pupils at all stages of their education. Technical innovations, such as voice recognition software and text-to-speech computer programs (described in Appendix D) are available to help dyslexic readers in education and in the workplace. Organisations such as the British Dyslexia Association, the European Dyslexia Association, and the International Dyslexia Association (see Appendix A) now provide a huge amount of information and support to individuals, families, and teachers.

Screening for dyslexia

The first stage in identifying whether someone is dyslexic usually starts with generalised screening for learning disorders. This screening will not identify a child as being dyslexic but it can identify those whose learning and behavioural problems suggest that they might be dyslexic. Screening is usually undertaken by a teacher or an educational psychologist. It is often carried out with large numbers of children, and usually takes the form of a checklist of questions (e.g.: www.amidyslexic.co.uk/am-i-dyslexic.html) or a few short tests of ability.

Screening checklists generally ask individuals about their:

- reading, e.g. when you read, do you often lose your place on the line?
- writing, e.g. is your writing difficult to read?
- spelling, e.g. do you sometimes spell a word in different ways on the same page?
- memory, e.g. do you have difficulty remembering telephone numbers while you dial?
- spoken language skills, e.g. when you say a long word, do you sometimes have difficulty saying all the sounds in the correct order?
- educational history, e.g. did you struggle to learn your multiplication tables at school?
- family history, e.g. do you have a family history of reading difficulties?
- problems confusing left and right, e.g. do you sometimes forget which way is left and which is right?
- difficulties with time-keeping, e.g. do you often arrive late for appointments or miss them altogether?

Answering 'yes' to more than a specified number of these questions is taken as a sign that a more thorough assessment may be warranted.

The most common screening (ability) tests are:

- The Bangor Dyslexia Test
- The Dyslexia Screening Test
- The Dyslexia Early Screening Test
- The Dyslexia Adult Screening Test
- Lucid Adult Dyslexia Screening
- Lucid Cognitive Profiling System
- Lucid Rapid Dyslexia Screening
- Pre-school Screening Test

- Quest
- Quickscan

These tests are summarised in Appendix C.

The use of screening tests can, of course, produce false positive results – individuals may be identified as being dyslexic when they are not – and false negative results – individuals may be deemed not to be dyslexic when they are. Therefore, care must be taken in drawing conclusions from these tests, particularly if the individual displays signs and symptoms of other developmental disorders that often occur alongside dyslexia, such as:

- poor motor skills and coordination (dyspraxia);
- poor concentration, inattention, and hyperactivity (ADHD);
- slow and messy handwriting (dysgraphia);
- difficulty with counting and with mental arithmetic (dyscalculia).

If the results of the screening test point to the existence of specific learning difficulties, the individual should be referred to a psychologist or specialist dyslexia teacher for a full diagnostic assessment.

Diagnostic assessment

Testing for dyslexia takes around two to three hours and involves a thorough assessment of the person's history, abilities, and attainment. Further details of the tests of cognitive ability, educational attainment and intellectual ability listed below may be found in Appendix C.

Background

A diagnosis of dyslexia is only made when reading and spelling difficulties cannot be readily explained by other factors. These might include poor hearing (which would impair the individual's awareness of the sounds of language), a disrupted education (the individual has not received enough reading instruction to enable them to read successfully), or insufficient experience of language (where the language spoken in school is/was different from the language spoken at home). So, questions will be asked about the individual:

- Medical history – e.g. were there any medical complications during their birth? Have they suffered from any serious illnesses or had any accidents involving head injuries?
- School history – e.g. have they had long periods of absence from school? How do they/did they feel about going to school?
- Family history – e.g. do any family members have reading, spelling, or language difficulties? How frequently has the family moved house, necessitating a change of school for the child?
- Speech and language history – e.g. at what age did they say their first words? What languages are spoken at home?
- Vision and hearing – e.g. do they have any uncorrected eyesight problems? Do they have problems with their hearing?

Cognitive ability

This includes assessment of language production and comprehension – particularly phonological processing ability – visual and auditory memory skills, and speed of information processing. Difficulty with any of these skills could indicate dyslexia.

Examples of cognitive ability tests that may be used are:

- The Phonological Assessment Battery
- The Phonological Abilities Test
- Comprehensive Tests of Phonological Processing
- The Wechsler Memory Scale

Educational attainment

This includes tests of single word reading and spelling, sentence reading and spelling, non-word reading, comprehension, handwriting, and tests of mathematical ability (to test for dyscalculia). The results of these tests provide an indication of the individual's 'basic skills' relative to those of others of the same age.

Examples of these tests are:

- The Edinburgh Reading Test
- The Graded Word Spelling Test
- The Gray Oral Reading Tests
- The Gray Silent Reading Tests
- The Listening and Literacy Index
- The Test of Word Reading Efficiency
- The Neale Analysis of Reading Ability
- The Wide Range Achievement Test
- The Woodcock Reading Mastery Test – Revised
- The Basic Number Screening Test
- Dyscalculia Screener

Intellectual ability

This includes measures of general verbal and non-verbal ability which provide an indication of intellectual potential. Someone with a high intellectual ability should perform well on all verbal and non-verbal tests. Someone with dyslexia is likely to show a less consistent intellectual profile, typically showing poorer performance on verbal tests than on non-verbal tests. If a discrepancy is found between actual educational attainment and attainment predicted by intellectual ability, this will indicate areas of specific educational difficulty.

The most commonly used tests of intellectual ability for children are:

- The Wechsler Intelligence Scale for Children
- The British Ability Scales (UK)/Differential Ability Scales (US)
- The Wide Range Intelligence Test

For adults, the following are commonly used:

- The Wechsler Adult Intelligence Scale
- The Wide Range Intelligence Test

A psychologist or specialist dyslexia teacher can use the results from these tests – together with results from the tests of educational attainment and cognitive ability, and information about the individual's background – to diagnose dyslexia and identify the individual's intellectual strengths and weaknesses. One dyslexic reader, Adrian, recalls when his performance on a battery of diagnostic tests was plotted on a graph:

> [A lady in the learning Support Unit] said 'Alright, now we'll put your scores on this', like a line, she said 'If you got a line you're normal'. And then mine were just like the Himalayas, so it was just like … 'What does that mean?' She said 'You're dyslexic'.
>
> *Dyslexia, the Self and Higher Education* by David Pollak, p. 193

This information – the high points on the graph representing strengths, as well as the low points representing weaknesses – can be used to design and implement an effective teaching strategy.

Managing dyslexia in schools

While there is always more that can be done to support and encourage dyslexic children in school, we have come a long way from the dyslexia-unaware days of thirty or more years ago. The author John Irving remembers this of his time at school:

> The diagnosis of dyslexia wasn't available in the late fifties – bad spelling like mine was considered a psychological problem by the language therapist who evaluated my mysterious case. When the repeated courses of language therapy were judged to have had no discernible influence on me, I was turned over to the school psychiatrist.

Today the schooling of children with special educational needs is increasingly covered by governmental regulations such as the Individuals with Disabilities Education Act (IDEA 2004) in the US, and by the Special Educational Needs Code of Practice (2001) in the UK. The introduction of laws to cover the identification and assessment of pupils with special educational needs has helped to bring about greater awareness of dyslexia, and of the need to provide appropriate educational, psychological, and technological support to dyslexic pupils both within and without mainstream education.

The following sections outline the stages involved in assessing and meeting the special educational needs of children with dyslexia in the United States and the United Kingdom.

Special education in the United States

In the US, children with specific learning difficulties are entitled to Special Education and Related Services tailored to their particular needs. For a child to gain access to these services a request for evaluation must first come from either the child, the parents, or the school. If the school agrees that the child has special educational needs then an evaluation will be undertaken. However, if the school disagrees, then they may refuse to undertake an evaluation. In this instance parents have the right of appeal against this decision and they may apply for an Independent Educational Evaluation of their child's needs.

Evaluation of a child's needs

An evaluation involves a full and comprehensive assessment of a child's needs for Special Education and Related Services. It may include an assessment of the child's general intelligence, communication skills, school performance, vision, hearing, and social and emotional well-being. Some of this information may be held by the school already, while some extra information may need to be collected at this stage. This information may be collected from:

- the child (although the written informed consent of the parents must be obtained before any additional testing is undertaken of the child);
- the child's parents;
- the child's classroom teachers;
- any special education teachers that have worked with the child;
- a school administrator – this person may be consulted regarding the general curriculum and resources available within, or available to, the school;
- an outside specialist who may help to interpret the results of the evaluation and to implement these in terms of the child's future schooling;
- any other outside specialists, such as school psychologists or speech and language therapists, as deemed necessary by the school or the parents.

Children with special educational needs must be re-evaluated on a regular basis, at least once every three years.

Eligibility for special education services

The information obtained through the course of the evaluation is used to determine the child's eligibility for special educational assistance. The final decision regarding eligibility is made by a group of individuals including the child's parents. If the decision is made that the child is not eligible, and the parents disagree with this decision, they retain the right to appeal against it. In this case parents should seek the advice of their state's Parent Training and Information Center.

Once a child has been identified as being eligible for Special Education and Related Services, an Individualized Education Program (an IEP) will be constructed specifically for the educational needs of that child.

Individualized Education Programs

The IEP is a written statement including information about:

- the child's current academic performance (their strengths and weaknesses);
- the child's particular educational needs;
- annual goals and objectives that will help to address these specific educational needs;
- details of how the child's progress towards these goals will be determined objectively;
- details of special circumstances or modifications that need to be in place to allow the child to participate in 'state and district-wide' tests of achievement;
- specialist support (e.g. dedicated teaching or assistive technology) that must be provided;
- how, where, when, and by whom this support will be provided.

At the heart of the IEP is the need for support which allows the dyslexic child to participate fully in the general curriculum, in the 'least restrictive environment'. The focus must be on inclusion rather than exclusion, so wherever possible the child will be taught alongside his or her peers in the general classroom. The relative success of the IEP will be reviewed on an annual basis (or more often if needed).

Special education in the United Kingdom

The UK Code of Practice identifies a three step approach to the teaching of children with special educational needs. For school-age children (as opposed to pre-school children, for whom the approach is very slightly different) these steps are called: (1) School Action, (2) School Action Plus, (3) Request for Statutory Assessment.

School Action

Teachers become aware that individual children are failing to progress with their reading. In response to this, they may provide additional teaching to address the child's particular weaknesses. If the child still fails to progress in their reading, the next step involves consultation between the teacher, the special educational needs coordinator (SENCO), and the child's parents to decide what extra provision is needed. This may involve bringing in extra teaching support, using specialist teaching materials or specialist equipment. During this process an Individual Education Plan (IEP) is written to specify the action that the school, the pupil, and the parents agree to take. This will include:

- short-term targets such as, 'by the end of this term, Jessica will have learned how to write the alphabet';

- possible strategies to be used by teachers, parents, and external specialists to help the child to achieve this target;
- criteria by which the IEP may be deemed to be a success or a failure;
- outcomes of these targets and strategies;
- the review date for the IEP.

The success of this plan is reviewed regularly.

If the child continues to make poor progress, in spite of having an IEP, or if it is decided that their particular educational needs cannot be met under the School Action plan, then step two – School Action Plus is implemented.

School Action Plus

At this stage the school consults an outside specialist – e.g. an educational psychologist – to assess the child's educational needs. A new IEP is written to identify a new plan of action for the child's education based on this assessment. Again, this is reviewed on a regular basis.

For some children, support provided as part of School Action Plus is not sufficient to meet their particular needs. In these cases, as long as it may be demonstrated that every effort has been made to meet the child's educational needs, a Statutory Assessment may be requested by the child's parents or teachers. If the request comes from the school, the parents must be informed of this.

Request for Statutory Assessment

Once the request has been made it is up to the Local Authority (LA) to decide whether or not to make the Statutory Assessment. The decision to go ahead with a Statutory Assessment will be made if the LA considers that the child's educational needs will be best met by the issuing of a Statement of Special Educational Needs. It should be noted that the call for a Statutory Assessment does not necessarily end with the issuing of a Statement.

Statements of Special Educational Needs

If the decision is made to go ahead with a Statutory Assessment, evidence of the child's educational and psychological needs may be requested by the LA from the parents, the school, from educational psychologists, Social Services, and any other outside specialist as appropriate. On the basis of this evidence, the LA may decide to issue a Statement of Special Educational Needs. This must include:

- details of the child's specific educational needs, with supporting evidence;
- specific information regarding how these needs will be met, with set objectives, details of provision, and how and when these arrangements should be reviewed;
- details of any non-educational needs that the child may have if they are to benefit from the specialist help detailed in the Statement;
- how these needs will be met.

Once a Statement has been made, the child's parents and all of his/her teachers must be informed of this, and the child's progress (i.e. the success of the Statement) must be reviewed at least once a year thereafter.

A hidden disability?

There has been some debate as to whether dyslexia should be considered to be a disability. Legally, a disability is defined as, 'a physical or mental impairment that substantially limits one or more major life activities' (the Americans with Disabilities Act, 1990), or 'a physical or mental impairment which has a substantial and long-term adverse effect on a person's ability to carry out normal day-to-day activities' (the UK Disability Discrimination Act, 1995).

In these definitions, 'physical impairment' might include weakening of any part of the body through illness or accident, blindness, deafness, paralysis, or heart disease, while 'mental impairment' might include depression and learning disabilities, such as dyslexia and dyspraxia. This impairment must be regarded as being more than a minor inconvenience – i.e. it must either increase the time that might normally be required to perform an activity, or it might actually preclude the performance of this activity. Finally, the activities affected by this impairment include everyday aspects of life that require mobility, manual dexterity, physical coordination, speech, hearing, eyesight, memory, and the ability to concentrate, learn, or understand. So, according to these definitions, severe dyslexia may be considered to be a disability, and dyslexic people cannot legally be discriminated against when applying for jobs or educational courses because of their reading difficulties.

Others have argued against the blanket description of dyslexia as a 'disability' as no two dyslexic readers experience precisely the same difficulties. It is only in certain situations that a person with dyslexia will be adversely affected by his/her reading impairments. Dyslexic readers, however severe their disorder, are often adept at covering up their difficulties during their years at school and in their professional lives. They tend to avoid situations in which they might have to read aloud, or to write things down, and they may choose to enter careers that minimise the need to read or write. Consider, for example, two people with dyslexia; one becomes a teacher while the other becomes a professional footballer. While the teacher will face difficulties every day relating to his/her impaired reading and writing, the footballer has no particular need to read or write so will face no such difficulties. So while both individuals are equally dyslexic, the teacher may well be considered to be disabled by their dyslexia, whereas the footballer may not.

Alternatively, consider another two people with dyslexia, one of whom is English while the other is Italian. As you saw in chapter 5, English is a complex, irregular language while Italian is a highly regular language. So while both individuals are dyslexic, the English speaker is likely to be disabled by his/her dyslexia whereas the Italian speaker may not even be aware that he/she has a reading difficulty. This problem of the English language has been described in the following way:

> In terms of the social model of disability, I have always regarded the brain functions associated with dyslexia as part of a perfectly normal variation in the population, but the English language as a social factor 'disabling' dyslexics in much the same way as stairs inhibit those in wheelchairs.
>
> *Dyslexia, the Self and Higher Education* by David Pollak, p. 149

Teaching dyslexic children in the classroom

Traditional classroom teaching involves vision and hearing – the teacher speaks and writes on the blackboard (or whiteboard) and perhaps shows pictures, while the children look and listen. As you can probably appreciate, this method of teaching is problematic for dyslexic children who may have difficulties with their vision (perhaps experiencing visual stress and glare from the room's fluorescent lights), with their phonological processing (their processing of rapid speech sounds), and with their verbal memory (remembering what has been said). So what can be done to accommodate the needs of the dyslexic child within the general classroom? In the words of Dr Harry Chasty, former director of the Dyslexia Institute (now, Dyslexia Action):

> If the child doesn't learn the way you teach, teach him the way he learns.

Research has shown that dyslexic readers (and non-dyslexic readers) learn best when they are taught using 'multi-sensory' teaching methods – i.e. teaching not only in the visual and auditory modalities but also in the tactile (touch) and kinaesthetic (movement) modalities. For example, when teaching young children to read, written letters may be linked to their corresponding sounds by the teacher showing the letter or string of letters (e.g. *tion*) while saying its sound ('shun'). The children may be encouraged to repeat the sound while making the shape of the letters with their hands or with their bodies. They may draw the letters in the air, shape them out of modelling clay or pipe-cleaners, or draw them onto sandpaper or the carpet. As a child sees letters, says their sounds and feels their shapes, the brain receives the same information simultaneously in different ways, creating a stronger multi-sensory memory.

Teaching using these methods is undertaken in a cumulative, sequential way, building from individual letters/letter strings, through single-syllable words to increasingly complex multi-syllabic words. Conditional letter-sound rules are also taught in a highly structured and explicit way. For example, if the letter 'g' is followed by an 'e', 'i', or 'y' it may be pronounced as a soft 'j' sound (as in *gentle*, *giant*, and *gymnasium*); if it is followed by any other letter it is pronounced as a hard 'g' sound (as in *garland*, *gold*, and *glad*). Children may be encouraged to produce words beginning with either the 'j' or the 'g' sound, using plastic letters to spell the words out. This approach helps dyslexic and non-dyslexic readers alike to learn the letter-sound relationships that underlie reading and spelling.

Other 'dyslexia-friendly' strategies in education

Dyslexic students of all ages need to be supported through their education, and there are numerous strategies that may be beneficial to these students whether at school, college, or university. In particular, the teacher/lecturer can:

- encourage dyslexic students to sit near the front of the class so that they may see and hear as clearly as possible;
- provide handouts/lecture notes where possible rather than requiring students to make their own notes during classes/lectures;
- outline the structure of the class/lecture clearly at the start;
- give dyslexic students permission to tape-record their classes/lectures;
- avoid embarrassing dyslexic students by asking them to read aloud in front of others;
- avoid the use of fluorescent lighting where possible;
- allow sufficient time for students to complete their written work;
- allow students to take short breaks during class;
- wherever possible, avoid presenting black text on a white background (e.g. using a black pen on a whiteboard or an overhead projector); using chalk and a blackboard instead will reduce glare;
- allow students to work on coloured paper;
- be careful not to present information on PowerPoint slides which have background images that distract the eye from the text;
- avoid the use of lecture slides or handouts that contain lots of text; these should include only key points;
- present information in bullet points rather than as continuous text;

- present information visually as much as possible;
- use a font of at least size 12 point in lecture notes and handouts;
- use a clear, sans-serif font (e.g. Arial or Verdana) that does not have the additional 'ticks' and 'strokes' that form part of the letters in a serif font (e.g. Times or Courier);
- left-align text on slides and handouts rather than justifying or centring it;
- use lower case text on lecture slides/handouts in preference to upper case text;
- use double-spacing (or at least 1.5) rather than single spacing;
- write anything that is particularly important (e.g. key terms) in capital letters;
- always make sure that dyslexic students understand what is required of them – i.e. that they understand the essay question or the nature of the assessment. This should be provided on a handout rather than requiring students to copy the title of the assignment from the board;
- try to avoid setting complex assessment questions that might easily be misread and misunderstood;
- try to develop methods of assessment that require little writing;
- encourage students to discuss their thoughts before they begin writing their assessed work;
- encourage dyslexic students to have someone read through their work for understanding before they hand it in;
- encourage students to affix dyslexia cover sheets/stickers (where these are used) to their assessed work so that the assessor will be aware that the work was done by a dyslexic student; the assessor should also be made aware of the particular errors that may be associated with dyslexia;
- make allowance for poor spelling when reading a dyslexic student's work;
- explain clearly to students where they went wrong, when

mistakes are made in written work, and how such mistakes could be avoided in the future;
- encourage and praise dyslexic students whenever possible to raise their self-esteem;
- encourage students to make use of language and learning support services that are available;
- encourage students to utilise assistive technology, such as speech recognition programs, essay-planning software (e.g. Inspiration) and to prepare their work on computer, making use of the spell check facility.

Many of the difficulties of dyslexia can be managed with appropriate teaching, support, and encouragement, and many dyslexic readers achieve academic success. According to one report, dyslexic readers who graduate from university achieve grades that do not differ significantly from those of their non-dyslexic peers (UK National Working Party on Dyslexia in Higher Education, 1999).

Dyslexia in the workplace

Many of the strategies suitable for helping dyslexic students in education can also be adopted in the workplace. For example, dyslexia-friendly employers can:

- provide a clear, written agenda before meetings, and written notes afterwards;
- allow sufficient time for the completion of projects;
- avoid asking dyslexic employees to read aloud in front of others;
- allow dyslexic employees to present their work on coloured paper;
- factor in frequent short breaks during long meetings;

- always make sure that dyslexic employees understand what is required of them – i.e. that they understand the nature of the assignment;
- provide assistive technology – e.g. computers with speech recognition software, text reading software, portable voice recorders – where appropriate;
- offer praise and encouragement where possible.

Dyslexia and entrepreneurship

Research conducted at London's Cass Business School – led by Professor Julie Logan – has shown that around 35% of entrepreneurs in the US and 19% in the UK are dyslexic. This contrasts with figures of 1% in the US and 3% in the UK amongst corporate managers (i.e. business managers who work for other people).

Relative to non-dyslexic entrepreneurs, those with dyslexia were found to be more likely to:

- be more creative;
- have excellent problem-solving skills;
- work in engineering and manufacturing;
- have a higher need to achieve;
- own more than one business;
- have started their own businesses immediately after leaving school;
- have developed their businesses more quickly;
- manage a greater number of staff;
- be more likely to delegate authority.

The authors of this study suggest that dyslexic readers' ability to think through problems in a creative way, to pursue their dreams in spite of the obstacles, to motivate others to share their vision, and to surround themselves with people whose skills compensate for their own difficulties, may reflect coping strategies that they have developed through their lives. These strategies help them to deal with the problems and uncertainties of living as a dyslexic reader in a non-dyslexic world; they might also endow significant numbers of dyslexic adults with an 'edge' in business.

The final word goes to US Congresswoman Carolyn McCarthy, herself dyslexic, who urges:

> Never let dyslexia be an excuse for not achieving success. Chart your course and work to make your dreams a reality. Once you do that, there is nothing to ever hinder you.

Further reading

Chapter 1

A number of excellent books describe the day-to-day experiences of children and adults with developmental dyslexia, including Abraham Schmitt's *Brilliant Idiot: An Autobiography of a Dyslexic* (1994, Intercourse, PA: Good Books); Lissa Weinstein's *Reading David: A Mother and Son's Journey Through the Labyrinth of Dyslexia* (2004, New York: Perigee Trade); Robert Frank and Kathryn Livingston's *Secret Life of a Dyslexic Child: How She Thinks. How He Feels. How They Can Succeed* (2004, Emmaus Press, PA: Rodale Press); John Osmond's *The Reality of Dyslexia* (1993, London: Cassell Education and Channel 4); Eileen Simpson's *Reversals. A Personal Account of Victory over Dyslexia* (1991, New York: The Noonday Press), and Joy Pollock, Elisabeth Waller, and Rody Politt's *Day-to-Day Dyslexia in the Classroom*, 2nd edition (2004, London: RoutledgeFalmer). An interesting article, 'Experiences of a sufferer from word-blindness', can be downloaded from the website of the *British Journal of Ophthalmology* (http://bjo.bmj.com/content/vo120/issue2/).

Some good books for dyslexic children to read are Diane Burton Robb's *The Alphabet War: A Story about Dyslexia* (2004, Morton Grove, IL: Albert Whitman & Company); Caroline Janover's *Josh: A Boy with Dyslexia* (2004, Lincoln, NE: iUniverse.com), and Henry Winkler and Lin Oliver's series of books about a ten-year-old dyslexic boy called Hank Zipzer (including *Niagara Falls – or does it?* and *I got a 'D' in salami* (London: Walker Books Ltd)). These books tell the story of fictional children with dyslexia – their reading difficulties, their emotional frustrations, and ways that they find to deal with their learning problems – and will help children to gain a better understand of their own dyslexia.

The following books are out of print but well worth seeking out in a library or second-hand bookshop: *Susan's Story: An Autobiographical Account of My Struggle with Words* (1982, New York: St Martin's Press) and *Every Letter Counts: Winning in Life Despite Dyslexia* (1990, London: Bantam Press) by Susan Hampshire; and Girard J. Sagmiller's *Dyslexia, My Life: One Man's Story of His Life with a Learning Disability* (2000, Lee's Summit, MO: DT Publishing).

Good books describing what life is like for young people and adults with dyslexia and dyspraxia are: David Grant's *That's the Way I Think: Dyslexia and Dyspraxia Explained* (2005, London: David Fulton Publishers Ltd) and Mary Colley's *Living with Dyspraxia: A Guide for Adults with Developmental Dyspraxia*, 4th edition (2006, London: Jessica Kingsley Publishers).

Chapter 2

An excellent book on the development of reading and spelling is Marilyn Jager Adams's *Beginning To Read: Thinking and Learning About Print* (1990, Cambridge, MA: MIT Press). Other good sources of information are Margaret Snowling and Charles Hulmes's *The Science of Reading. A Handbook* (2005, Oxford: Blackwell Publishing Ltd); Jane Oakhill and Alan Garnham's *Becoming a Skilled Reader* (1988, Oxford: Blackwell Publishing Ltd); Geoffrey Underwood and Vivienne Batt's *Reading and Understanding* (1996, Oxford: Blackwell Publishing Ltd); and Keith Rayner and Alexander Pollatsek's *The Psychology of Reading.* (1994, London: Lawrence Erlbaum Associates). Andrew Ellis's *Reading, Writing and Dyslexia: A*

Cognitive Analysis, 2nd edition (1993, Hove: Lawrence Erlbaum) gives an easy-to-read introduction to the processes underlying normal and impaired reading development.

The teaching of reading, and the importance of phonics in reading development, are covered by the following: Usha Goswami and Peter Bryant's *Phonological Skills and Learning to Read* (1990, Hove: Lawrence Erlbaum); Terezinha Nunes and Peter Bryant's *Handbook of Children's Literacy* (2003, Dordrecht: Kluwer Academic Publishers); Jane Oakhill and Roger Beard's *Reading Development and the Teaching of Reading: A Psychological Perspective* (1999, Oxford: Blackwell Publishers Ltd); and Keith Rayner and colleagues' (2002) article, 'How should reading be taught?' in *Scientific American*, March, 84–91. Claire Jamieson and Juliet Jamieson's *Manual for Testing and Teaching English Spelling* (2003, Chichester: John Wiley and Sons Ltd) provides a useful guide to the teaching of spelling to dyslexic and non-dyslexic readers, and to those learning English as an additional language.

The 'Rose report' – *Independent Review of the Teaching of Early Reading: Final Report* (2006) – is available from: www.standards. dfes.gov.uk/phonics/report.pdf.

Chapter 3

An excellent summary of the phonological model of dyslexia can be found in Sally Shaywitz's (1996) article 'Dyslexia' in *Scientific American*, November, 98–104; Valerie Muter's *Early Reading Development and Dyslexia* (2003, London: Whurr Publishers); Usha Goswami and Peter Bryant's *Phonological Skills and Learning to Read* (1990, Hove: Lawrence Erlbaum); and Janet Hatcher and Margaret Snowling's chapter in Reid and Wearmouth's *Dyslexia and Literacy* (2002, Chichester: John Wiley and Sons Ltd).

A good book that highlights ways in which phonological difficulties may be tackled in the teaching of dyslexic children is Margaret Walton's *Teaching Reading and Spelling to Dyslexic Children: Getting to Grips with Words* (1998, London: David Fulton Publishers Ltd).

A less serious take on the phonological difficulties associated with dyslexia is Roald Dahl's *The Vicar of Nibbleswicke* (1992, London: Penguin Books) – about a vicar whose 'Back-to-Front' dyslexia causes him to speak words backwards. Dahl wrote this to raise funds for the Dyslexia Institute (now, Dyslexia Action).

Chapter 4

A good introduction to visual processes in dyslexia can be found in: John Everatt's *Reading and Dyslexia: Visual and Attentional Processes* (1999, London: Routledge); Bruce Evans's *Dyslexia and Vision* (2001, Philadelphia, PA: Whurr Publishers); and Alan Beaton's *Dyslexia, Reading and the Brain: A Sourcebook of Psychological and Biological Research* (2004, Hove: Psychology Press). For an overview of eye movements during reading see Keith Rayner et al.'s chapter in Snowling and Hulme's *The Science of Reading. A Handbook* (2005, Oxford: Blackwell).

Good books on visual stress and the use of colour lenses to alleviate visual stress in dyslexia are Arnold Wilkins' *Reading through Colour* (2003, Chichester: John Wiley and Sons); Helen Irlen's *Reading by the Colors. Overcoming Dyslexia and Other Reading Disabilities through the Irlen Method*, revised edition (2005, New York: Perigee Books); and Rhonda Stone's *The Light Barrier: A Color Solution to Your Child's Light-Based Reading Difficulties* (2002, New York: St Martin's Press).

For an overview of the link between dyslexia and visual strength/creativity see Thomas West's *In the Mind's Eye* (1997, Amherst, NY: Prometheus Books); Beverly Steffert's chapter in

S. Dingli's *Creative Thinking: Towards Broader Horizons* (1998, Msida: Malta University Press); Catya von Károlyi et al.'s (2003) article, 'Dyslexia linked to talent: Global visual-spatial ability', in *Brain and Language*, 85, 427–431; and Ulrika Wolff and Ingvar Lundberg's (2002) article, 'The prevalence of dyslexia among art students', in *Dyslexia*, 8, 1, 34–42.

Chapter 5

For further information on reading in different languages, see Julie Fiez's (2000) article, 'Sound and meaning: How native language affects reading strategies' in *Nature Neuroscience*, 3, 1, 3–5; Johannes Ziegler and Usha Goswami's (2006) article, 'Becoming literate in different languages: similar problems, different solutions' in *Developmental Science*, 9, 429–453; and Philip Seymour's chapter on early reading development in European orthographies in Snowling and Hulme's *The Science of Reading. A Handbook* (2005, Oxford: Blackwell). This topic is also covered in depth in Nicola Brunswick, Siné McDougall, and Paul de Mornay Davies's forthcoming book *The Role of Orthographies in Reading and Spelling* (in press, London: Psychology Press).

For excellent sources of information on dyslexia across different languages, see Taeko Wydell and Brian Butterworth's (1999) article, 'An English-Japanese bilingual with monolingual dyslexia' in *Cognition*, 70, 273–305; Eraldo Paulesu et al.'s (2001) article, 'Dyslexia: cultural diversity and biological unity' in *Science*, 291, 5511, 2165–2167; Markéta Caravolas's chapter on the nature and causes of dyslexia in different languages in Snowling and Hulme's *The Science of Reading. A Handbook* (2005, Oxford: Blackwell); Nata Goulandris's *Dyslexia in Different Languages: Cross-Linguistic Comparisons* (2003, London: Whurr Publishers); and Asher and Martin Hoyles's *Dyslexia from a Cultural Perspective* (2007, London: Hansib Publishing [Caribbean] Ltd). *Language Shock – Dyslexia across Cultures*, can be downloaded free in English, French, German, Spanish, and Portuguese from http://ditt-online.org/E-books.htm.

Chapter 6

Many excellent books and journal articles describe the brain's role in language. For example, David Sousa's *How the Brain Learns to Read* (2004, Thousand Oaks, CA: Corwin Press); Maryanne Wolf's *Proust and the Squid: The Story and Science of the Reading Brain* (2007, New York: HarperCollins Publishers); Julie Fiez and Steven Petersen's (1998) article, 'Neuroimaging studies of word reading', in *Proceedings of the National Academy of Sciences USA*, 95, 914–921; Morton Gernsbacher and Michael Kaschak's (2003) article, 'Neuroimaging studies of language production and comprehension' in *Annual Review of Psychology*, 54, 91–114; Peter Turkeltaub et al.'s (2003) article, 'Development of neural mechanisms for reading' in *Nature Neuroscience*, 6, 6, 767–773; and a special issue of *Cognition* on 'Towards a new functional anatomy of language', 2004, 92, 1–2.

For further reading on the processing of spoken and written language in dyslexia, see Jean-François Démonet et al.'s (2004) article, 'Developmental dyslexia' in *The Lancet*, 363, 1451–1460; Michel Habib's (2000) article, 'The neurological basis of developmental dyslexia' in *Brain*, 123, 2373–2399; M. Eckert's (2004) article, 'Neuroanatomical markers for dyslexia: A review of dyslexia structural imaging studies' in *The Neuroscientist*, 10, 4, 362–371; Nicola Brunswick's (2004) chapter, 'Developmental dyslexia: Evidence from brain research' in T. Nunes and P. Bryant's *Handbook of Literacy* (Dordrecht: Kluwer Press); and Nicola Brunswick and Neil Martin's (2006) chapter on the neuropsychology of language and language disorders in G.N. Martin, *Human Neuropsychology*, 2nd edition (Harlow: Prentice Hall).

Chapter 7

Although book chapters and articles on the genetics of language and dyslexia are not always for the faint-hearted, the following provide an interesting and readable introduction to the topic: Sebastian Haesler's (2007) article, 'Programmed for speech' in *Scientific American Mind*, 18, 3, 66–71; Richard Olson's 2005 Norman Geschwind memorial lecture on 'Genes, environment, and dyslexia', reproduced in the *Annals of Dyslexia*, 56, 2, 205–238; Elena Grigorenko's article on 'Developmental dyslexia: an update on genes, brains, and environments' in the *Journal of Child Psychology and Psychiatry and Allied Disciplines*, 42, 1, 91–125; Frank Ramus's (2004) 'Neurobiology of dyslexia: A reinterpretation of the data' in *Trends in Neuroscience*, 27, 12, 720–726; Bruce Pennington and Richard Olsen's (2005) chapter on the genetics of dyslexia in M. Snowling and C. Hulmes's *The Science of Reading. A Handbook* (Oxford: Blackwell Publishing Ltd); and Alan Beaton's chapter on the genetic background of dyslexia in his book, *Dyslexia, Reading and the Brain: A Sourcebook of Psychological and Biological Research* (2004, Hove: Psychology Press).

Chapter 8

Many good books have been written for families and teachers of those with dyslexia. These include: Philomena Ott's *How to Detect and Manage Dyslexia: A Reference and Resource Manual* (1997, Oxford: Heinemann Educational Publishers); Chris Neanon's *How to Identify and Support Children with Dyslexia*

(2002, London: LDA); Bevé Hornsby's *Overcoming Dyslexia: A Straightforward Guide for Families and Teachers*, 3rd edition (1996, London: Vermilion); Sally Raymond's *Helping Children Cope with Dyslexia*, 2nd edition (2002, London: Sheldon Press); Gavin Reid and Shannon Green's *100 Ideas for Supporting Pupils with Dyslexia* (2007, London: Continuum International Publishing Group Ltd); Jenny Cogan and Mary Flecker's *Dyslexia in Secondary School: A Practical Handbook for Teachers, Parents and Students* (2004, Chichester: John Wiley & Sons); and Bernice Baumer's *How to Teach Your Dyslexic Child to Read: A Proven Method for Parents and Teachers* (1998, Secaucus, NJ: Citadel Press). Ellen Morgan and Cynthia Klein's book, *The Dyslexic Adult in A Non-Dyslexic World* (2000, London: Whurr Publishers) is a good source of information and advice for anyone who lives with or works with dyslexic adults.

Julie Bennett's *Dyslexia Pocketbook* (2006, Alresford, UK: Teachers' Pocketbooks) provides many hints, tips, and techniques for helping dyslexic readers to achieve their potential, while Sandra Hargreaves's book, *Study Skills for Dyslexic Students* (2007, London: Sage Publications Ltd) includes a CD-ROM containing invaluable tools and resources for dyslexic students in further and higher education.

For practical advice on the teaching of number skills to dyslexic readers, see Pauline Clayton's *How to Develop Numeracy in Children with Dyslexia* (2003, London: LDA); Julie Kay and Dorian Yeo's *Dyslexia and Maths* (2003, London: David Fulton Publishers Ltd); and Anne Henderson's *Maths for the Dyslexic: A Practical Guide* (1998, London: David Fulton Publishers Ltd).

The British Dyslexia Association's *Dyslexia Handbook* is published annually and includes a great deal of information on the identification of dyslexia, sources of support, practical suggestions and advice for dyslexic readers at home, at school, in further and higher education, and in the workplace.

Glossary

ACID profile   A pattern of difficulties (poor performance on the Arithmetic, Coding, Information, and Digit span subtests of the WISC) believed by some to characterise dyslexia

Acquired dyslexia   A reading impairment that results from brain injury in individuals with previously normal reading ability

ADHD   Attention deficit/hyperactivity disorder; a developmental disorder that often co-occurs with dyslexia, characterised by poor concentration, inattention and hyperactivity

Analytic phonics   A process of reading instruction whereby children initially learn to read a set of whole words by sight. They are then taught to break these words down into their constituent parts and to explore ways in which words that share the same sounds also often share written letters

Assistive technology   Adaptive devices and products, including hardware and software, designed to assist dyslexic readers in their daily lives

Auditory discrimination   The ability to distinguish between sounds

Auditory (verbal) memory   The ability to recall lists of numbers or words presented verbally

Automaticity   The ability to perform a task without the need for conscious effort or attention

Binocular vision   A combination of the visual images from the two eyes that enables us to perceive depth and distance

Binocular convergence   Bringing the two eyes to converge steadily on a single spot

Blending   Combining individual sounds (parts of words) into a single spoken word (e.g. blending the sounds 'd', 'o', 'g' to produce the word *dog*)

Broca's area   A region of the brain in the frontal lobe, on the left side, associated with language production

Cerebellum   Part of the brain located at the back of the head, beneath the cerebral cortex, associated with movement, posture, and balance

Chronological age   An individual's age, usually expressed in years and months

Compensatory strategy   A procedure that may be adopted to help the individual to cope with his or her specific learning difficulties

Comprehension   Understanding of spoken or written language

Cone cells   Cells in the eye that enable us to see colour; found mainly in and around the fovea

Decoding   The process of converting written words into spoken language

Developmental dyslexia   An impairment in the development of reading and spelling skills that is not due to low intelligence or lack of educational opportunity

Diagnostic assessment   In-depth evaluation of an individual's cognitive strengths and weaknesses to test for the presence of specific learning difficulties such as dyslexia

Dyscalculia   A developmental disorder characterised by difficulty with numbers, counting, and performing mental arithmetic; it often co-occurs with dyslexia

Dysgraphia   A developmental disorder characterised by poor hand-eye coordination, difficulty performing fine motor tasks, and messy handwriting; it often co-occurs with dyslexia

Dyspraxia (developmental coordination disorder)   A developmental disorder characterised by poor motor skills, balance and coordination; it often co-occurs with dyslexia

Ectopias   Microscopic irregularities seen post-mortem in the language areas of some dyslexic brains. These irregularities disrupt the structure of the brain

Educational psychologist   A psychologist who specialises in the cognitive, social, and emotional development of children as this relates to teaching and learning

Essential fatty acids   Fatty acids (such as omega-3) which are essential for the normal development and function of the brain, and for the effective functioning of the immune system

Fixation stability   The stability of the eyes during visual fixation

Fovea   The centre of the retina; visual information that falls on the fovea is sharply focused

Frontal lobe   The region of cerebral cortex located at the front of the brain, associated with personality and forward planning; includes the motor cortex (and Broca's area)

Grapheme   A written letter or cluster of letters that correspond to a spoken phoneme

Grapheme-phoneme conversion   Converting written letters into their corresponding spoken sounds

Gyri   The 'bumps' on the surface of the brain

Homographs   Words that have the same spelling but different meanings; for example, the word *present*, which may be used as a noun ('the birthday *present* was given to the child') or a verb ('she was invited to *present* her argument')

Homophones   Words that are pronounced the same but have different meanings and spellings; for example, the words *birth* and *berth*

Individual Education Plan (UK)/Individualized Education Program (US)   A written statement specifying the particular educational needs of an individual pupil, the action that will be taken by parents, teachers, and other specialists to meet these needs, and the criteria by which this action may be deemed to be successful

Intelligence   Intellectual ability; may be expressed as verbal intelligence, non-verbal intelligence, or general intelligence (verbal plus non-verbal intelligence)

Irregular words   Words (such as *pint* and *yacht*) that do not conform to the most common letter-sound patterns of the language

Kinaesthetic   Pertaining to the movement of the muscles

Learning style   An individual's usual, and preferred, way of processing information

Lexical priming effect   Words that have been 'primed' are subsequently read faster than words that have not been primed

Lexical (semantic) reading   Reading by 'looking up' known, whole words in the mental lexicon; unknown words will not be read this way

Light sensitivity (also known as Meares-Irlen syndrome, scotopic sensitivity syndrome or visual stress)   Visual discomfort caused by bright (usually fluorescent) light, contrast, or glare; often causes eye strain and migraine headaches

Logograph   A written letter or symbol that represents an entire word without providing any indication of its pronunciation

Look-say reading   A method of reading whereby children learn to recognise whole words without decoding them

Magnocells   Large cells in the thalamus which detect orientation, movement, direction, and depth

Mental lexicon   A mental store of words and their meanings, like a 'mental dictionary'

Multi-sensory teaching   Teaching involving a combination of the visual, auditory, tactile, and kinaesthetic modalities

Occipital lobe   The region of cerebral cortex located at the back of the brain, associated with visual processing

Onset   The first part of a word that precedes the vowel (e.g. the 't' in the word *table*)

Orthographic depth   The complexity of the spelling-sound rules of a language; irregular languages are described as being deep or opaque, while regular languages are described as being shallow or transparent

Orthography   The rules of written language

Parietal lobe   The region of the cerebral cortex located behind the frontal lobe and above the temporal lobe, associated with visuospatial and sensory processing; includes the sensory cortex (and Wernicke's area)

Parvocells   Small cells in the thalamus which detect colour and fine detail

Phoneme   The smallest unit of sound that conveys meaning in speech (e.g. the word *cat* consists of the phonemes 'c', 'a', 't')

Phonics   A method of reading instruction that emphasises spelling-sound relationships

Phonological awareness   An understanding of the sound structure of spoken language

Planum temporale   A band of nerve fibres that connects the left and right hemispheres of the brain

Prefix   Letter strings such as 'un' and 'dis' that may be attached to the beginning of words to change their meaning

Pseudo-homophone   A legally spelt non-word that is intended to be pronounced in the same way as a real word, for example, *focks* and *gurl*

Pseudo-word   A string of letters that is pronounceable, but which has no meaning (e.g. *glomp*)

Rapid naming   The timed naming of visually presented objects, numbers, or colours, taken as an index of processing speed

Rate of articulation   The speed at which individuals are able to repeat words

Reading age   An indication of reading ability, usually expressed in years and months (e.g. a typically developing twelve-year-old child would be expected to have a reading age equivalent to, or slightly in excess of, twelve years)

Regular words   Words (such as *hand* and *string*) that conform to the most common letter-sound patterns of the language

Rhyme   The sharing of final phonemes but not necessarily graphemes (e.g. *meet/feet*, and *peat/suite*)

Rime   The final part of a word, including the first vowel and succeeding letters (e.g. 'able' in the word *table*)

Rod cells   Cells in the eye that enable us to see in dim light; found mainly around the outer edges of the retina

Saccade   A sudden, jerky movement of the eyes from one fixation point to another, such as when reading

Screening   The preliminary identification of signs and symptoms of a disorder, often by means of a checklist; may be followed by a full diagnostic assessment if the screening indicates that this is necessary

Semantics   Study of the meanings of words

Sequencing   The ordering of information (e.g. numbers, the months of the year, or multiplication tables) according to pre-determined rules

Short-term memory   A memory store that is limited in its capacity and duration

Sight vocabulary   Familiar words which an individual is able to recognise by sight without grapheme-phoneme decoding

Special educational needs coordinator (SENCO)   A teacher who is trained in the support of children with special educational needs, and who is responsible for the implementation and coordination of a school's special educational needs policy

Specific learning difficulties (SpLD)   A class of developmental disorders including dyslexia, dyspraxia, and ADHD which adversely affect an individual's ability to learn

Statement of Special Educational Needs   A statement issued by a Local Authority (LA) in the UK, following a statutory assessment, which identifies a child's specific educational needs, and the support that is required to meet those needs

Statutory assessment   If a child's particular educational needs cannot be met by his/her school, a detailed investigation of his/her needs (a statutory assessment) may be carried out by the LA;

this may (or may not) lead to the issuing of a Statement of Special Educational Needs

Sub-lexical (phonological) reading   Reading by converting the letters within words into their constituent sounds; irregular words will not be read correctly this way

Suffix   Letter strings such as 'ful' and 'able' that may be attached to the end of words to change their meaning

Sulci   The 'grooves' in the surface of the brain

Syntax   The grammatical rules of language

Synthetic phonics   A process of reading instruction whereby children are initially taught the sounds of the spoken language before being taught how to put these sounds together to form real words

Temporal lobe   The region of the cerebral cortex located beneath the frontal and parietal lobes, associated with the processing of language

Testosterone   The male sex hormone

Thalamus   A structure deep inside the brain that receives sensory information and passes it on to the part of the brain specialised to analyse it

Visual discrimination   The ability to distinguish between written symbols (shapes, letters, or numbers)

Visual field   When we look forwards, everything that we can see without moving our eyes, from the furthest point to our left to the further point to our right, from the furthest point above us to the furthest point below us

Visual memory   The ability to recall visual images (words, symbols, or objects)

Visual tracking   Following a moving target with the eyes

Visuospatial ability   The ability to process visual images and the spatial relationships between objects

WAIS   The Wechsler Adult Intelligence Scale – an intelligence test for adults

Wernicke's area   A region of the brain, on the left side, associated with language comprehension

WISC   The Wechsler Intelligence Scale for Children – an intelligence test for children

Working memory   A short-term memory store in which information may be retained and processed at the same time

Appendix A

Support organisations

The following organisations are excellent sources of information, support, and resources for children and adults with dyslexia, and their families:

British Dyslexia Association

Unit 8, Bracknell Beeches, Bracknell, RG12 7BW, UK. Tel: +44 (0)845 251 9003. Helpline: +44 (0)845 251 9002; email: helpline@bdadyslexia.org.uk; website: www.bdadyslexia.org.uk/

Canadian Dyslexia Association

207 Bayswater Avenue, Ottawa, Ontario, K1Y 2G5, Canada. Tel: +1 613 722 2699; email: info@dyslexiaassociation.ca; website: www.dyslexiaassociation.ca/

Dyslexia Action

Park House, Wick Road, Egham, Surrey, TW20 0HH, UK. Tel: +44 (0)1784 222 300; email: info@dyslexiaaction.org.uk; website: www.dyslexiaaction.org.uk/

Dyslexia Association of Ireland

Suffolk Chambers, 1 Suffolk Street, Dublin 2, Ireland. Tel: +353 (0)1 679 0276; email: info@dyslexia.ie; website: www.dyslexia.ie/index.htm

Dyslexia Scotland

Stirling Business Centre, Wellgreen, Stirling, FK8 2DZ, UK. Tel: +44 (0)844 800 8484; email: info@dyslexiascotland.org.uk; www.dyslexiascotland.org.uk/

European Dyslexia Association

www.dyslexia.eu.com/index.html

International Dyslexia Association

40 York Road, 4th Floor, Baltimore, MD 21204, USA. Tel: +1 410 296 0232; website: www.interdys.org

International Reading Association

800 Barksdale Road, P.O. Box 8139, Newark, DE 19714–8139, USA. Tel: +1 800 336 7323 (from US and Canada) +1 302 731 1600 (from elsewhere); email: pubinfo@reading.org; website: www.reading.org/

Northern Ireland Dyslexia Association

17a Upper Newtownards Road, Belfast, BT4 3HT, UK. Tel: +44 (0)28 9065 9212; email: help@nida.org.uk; website: www.nida.org.uk/

Appendix B

Journals

Annals of Dyslexia

An interdisciplinary, peer-reviewed journal published biannually by the International Dyslexia Association (IDA). Publishes original research articles on dyslexia and its associated conditions, remediation, and intervention. Members of the IDA receive free online access to this journal; printed copies are available to members for $15 per year. Website: www.springer.com/linguistics/languages+&+literature/journal/11881

Brain and Language

An interdisciplinary, peer-reviewed journal published twelve times a year. Publishes original research articles on the neurobiological basis of language. A personal subscription to the journal costs $707 (within the US) or €877 (across Europe). Website: www.elsevier.com/wps/find/journalbibliographicinfo.cws_home/622799/description?navopenmenu=-2

British Journal of Educational Psychology

A peer-reviewed journal published four times a year by the British Psychological Society. Publishes empirical (research), theoretical, and methodological articles on language, literacy, numeracy, and learning, including developmental disorders. A personal subscription to the journal costs £45 (within the UK), €67 (across Europe), or $83 (within the US). Website: www. bpsjournals.co.uk/journals/bjep/

Dyslexia

An interdisciplinary, peer-reviewed journal published four times a year in association with the British Dyslexia Association (BDA). Publishes original research articles and theoretical reviews on dyslexia, its assessment, and intervention. A personal subscription costs £50 for BDA members, or £75 for non-members. Website: www3.interscience.wiley.com/journal/6124/home/ProductInformation.html

Journal of Educational Psychology

An interdisciplinary, peer-reviewed journal published quarterly by the American Psychological Association. Publishes original research articles on aspects of education across all ages and levels. A personal subscription to this journal costs $161 within the US or $195 elsewhere. Website: www.apa.org/journals/edu/

Journal of Reading and Writing

An interdisciplinary, peer-reviewed journal published nine times a year, with empirical and theoretical articles on reading, writing, and spelling in English and other languages, and on developmental and acquired dyslexia. Members of the IDA receive free online access to this journal. Website: www. springer.com/linguistics/languages+&+literature/journal/11145

Perspectives on Language and Literacy

A journal published quarterly by the IDA. Publishes practical articles on the identification and management of dyslexia and its related disorders. Members of the IDA receive this journal free of charge; copies are available to non-members for $60 per year within the US or $99 elsewhere. Website: www.interdys. org/Perspectives.htm

Reading Psychology

An international, peer-reviewed journal published five times a year. Publishes original research articles on literacy and reading by children and adults. A personal subscription is available for £157 ($260/€208). Website: www.tandf.co.uk/journals/tf/ 02702711.html

Reading Research Quarterly

An interdisciplinary, peer-reviewed journal published quarterly by the International Reading Association (IRA). Publishes original research articles, theoretical, and methodological articles, on the teaching and learning of reading. Personal subscriptions are available to members of the IRA only, for $69. Website: www.reading.org/publications/journals/rrq/index.html

Scientific Studies of Reading

A peer-reviewed journal published quarterly by the Society for the Scientific Study of Reading. Publishes original research articles on all aspects of reading and writing by children and adults. A personal subscription to the journal costs £41 ($69/€55). Website: www.tandf.co.uk/journals/titles/10888438.asp

Appendix C
Tests for dyslexia

Dyslexia screening tests
The Bangor Dyslexia Test (BDT)

A test for individuals aged eight and over. It examines verbal repetition ability, working memory, sequencing ability, mental arithmetic, letter confusion, knowledge of times tables, handedness, and family history.

Dyslexia Early Screening Test (DEST-2)

A test for children aged four-and-a-half years to six-and-a-half years. It examines rapid naming, phonological awareness, working memory, sequencing, vocabulary, postural stability, and manual dexterity.

The Dyslexia Screening Test – Junior (DST-J)

A test for children aged six-and-a-half years to eleven-and-a-half years. It examines reading ability, spelling ability, rapid naming ability, phonological awareness, working memory, verbal fluency, vocabulary, postural stability, and manual dexterity.

Dyslexia Screening Test – Secondary (DST-S)

A test for children aged eleven-and-a-half years to sixteen-and-a-half years. It examines reading, writing, spelling, rapid naming, phonological awareness, working memory, verbal fluency, semantic fluency, non-verbal reasoning, postural stability, and manual dexterity.

Dyslexia Adult Screening Test (DAST)

A test for adults aged sixteen-and-a-half years plus. It examines reading, writing, spelling, rapid naming, phonological awareness, non-word reading, working memory, verbal fluency, semantic fluency, non-verbal reasoning, and postural stability.

Each of the above tests take about thirty minutes to complete.

Lucid Adult Dyslexia Screening (LADS)

A computer-based screening test for college and university students aged sixteen years plus. It examines phonological processing ability, working memory, word recognition, and non-verbal reasoning and takes around twenty minutes to complete.

Lucid Cognitive Profiling System (CoPS)

This is a computer-based screening test for children aged four to eight years. It examines phonological awareness, phoneme discrimination, auditory memory, visual memory, visual, and verbal sequencing. It takes around forty-five minutes to complete.

Lucid Rapid Dyslexia Screening

A computer-based screening test for children aged four to fifteen years. It examines phonological processing ability, working memory, phonic decoding skills, and visual-verbal memory. It takes around fifteen minutes to complete.

Pre-school Screening Test (PREST)

A test for children aged three-and-a-half years to four-and-a-half years. It examines repetition, rapid naming, shape copying, digits and letters, visual memory, and manual dexterity, and takes ten to fifteen minutes to complete. Children identified as being 'at risk' on the basis of initial screening may be tested further for phonological awareness, verbal memory, sequencing, visual matching, and postural stability. This takes a further ten to fifteen minutes.

Quest

A quick screening test and a more thorough diagnostic test for children aged six to eight years. It examines auditory and visual discrimination, auditory memory, visual sequencing, sight vocabulary, letter recognition, reading comprehension, and visuo-motor coordination. It takes around 30 minutes to complete.

Quickscan

A computer-based screening test for individuals aged sixteen years plus. It consists of approximately one hundred questions to examine learning style, reading ability, spelling ability, sequencing ability, memory, organisation, left–right awareness, hand–eye coordination, and family history. It takes around twenty minutes to complete.

Tests of cognitive ability

The Phonological Assessment Battery (PhAB)

A test that examines:

- alliteration – e.g. which two words, out of three presented orally, begin with the same sound?
- naming speed – picture naming and digit naming;
- rhyme – e.g. which two words, out of three presented orally, sound the same?

- spoonerisms – e.g. swap over the first sounds of the words *car* and *sad*;
- semantic fluency – e.g. name as many animals as you can;
- alliteration fluency – e.g. name as many words as you can that start with a 'p' sound;
- rhyme fluency – e.g. name as many words as you can that rhyme with *park*;
- non-word reading.

The Phonological Abilities Test (PAT)

A test that examines:

- rhyme detection – e.g. which of the words *door*, *tree*, or *lark* rhymes with *park*?
- rhyme production – e.g. say as many words as you can that rhyme with *bell*;
- word completion – e.g. here is a picture of a window; if I say the first part of the word ('win'), you say the last part ('doe'). Here is a picture of a match; if I say the first part of the word ('ma'), you say the last part ('tch');
- phoneme deletion – e.g. say the word *car* without the first sound, and the word *ball* without the last sound;
- letter knowledge;
- speech rate – e.g. say the word *buttercup* ten times as fast as you can.

Comprehensive Tests of Phonological Processing (CTOPP)

A test that examines:

- sound elision – e.g. say the word *crane* without the 'r' sound;
- blending words – e.g. what word is made when you put together the sounds 'd', 'o', 'g'?
- memory for spoken digits;

- non-word repetition;
- rapid naming of digits, letters, objects, and colours;
- blending non-words – e.g. what word is made when you put together the sounds 'f', 'i', 'p'?
- phoneme reversal – e.g. say *moof* backwards;
- segmenting words – e.g. say *milk* one sound at a time;
- segmenting non-words – e.g. say *glom* one sound at a time.

The Wechsler Memory Scale

A test that examines:

- immediate memory – e.g. listening to a list of numbers and repeating them immediately;
- delayed memory – e.g. listening to a list of numbers and repeating them after a delay;
- working memory – e.g. remembering a list of mixed letters and numbers and repeating them with the letters in alphabetical order and the numbers in numerical order;
- visual spatial span – e.g. remembering a visually presented sequence and reproducing it by tapping the sequence out on a series of blocks.

Tests of educational attainment

The Edinburgh Reading Test

A series of tests that assess vocabulary, syntax, sequencing, comprehension, skim reading, and the ability to 'read for facts'.

The Graded Word Spelling Test

A spelling test consisting of eighty words of increasing difficulty – from *in* and *am* to *abscess* and *menagerie* – each presented in the context of a sentence.

The Gray Oral Reading Tests (GORT)

A reading test that assesses reading rate, reading accuracy, and comprehension of passages of text of increasing difficulty.

The Gray Silent Reading Tests (GSRT)

An assessment of reading comprehension – individuals silently read passages of text of increasing difficulty and answer questions based on those passages.

The Listening and Literacy Index

A test of reading comprehension, listening comprehension, and spelling.

The Test of Word Reading Efficiency (TOWRE)

A test of sight word reading and non-word reading.

The Neale Analysis of Reading Ability (NARA II)

A test of reading rate, reading accuracy, and comprehension. Diagnostic information is provided about the individual's reading difficulties, with tests of the discrimination of first and last sounds, awareness of the names and sounds of letters, spelling ability, silent reading and writing ability, auditory discrimination, and the ability to blend sounds.

The Wide Range Achievement Test (WRAT-4)

A test that examines:

- reading – letter naming and the reading of single words of increasing difficulty;
- spelling – the writing of individual letters and words of increasing difficulty;

- arithmetic – counting, reading written numbers, mental arithmetic, and written arithmetic;
- sentence comprehension – comprehending ideas and information from whole sentences.

The Woodcock Reading Mastery Test-Revised (WRMT-R)

A test that examines:

- sight word reading;
- non-word reading – phonetic decoding efficiency;
- word comprehension – using tests requiring the identification of antonyms, synonyms, and analogies;
- passage comprehension – the individual reads a passage of text and then writes in words to complete sentences based on the text.

The Basic Number Screening Test

A test that assesses counting ability, the ability to write numbers and to do simple addition and subtraction

Dyscalculia Screener

A computer-based test that examines:

- dot enumeration – e.g. does the number of dots presented on the computer screen match the digit presented next to them?
- number comparison – e.g. which of two visually presented numbers is, numerically, larger?
- arithmetic achievement – e.g. simple addition and multiplication.

Tests of intellectual ability

The Wechsler Intelligence Scale for Children (WISC-IV)

The British Ability Scales (BAS) in the UK/Differential Ability Scales (DAS) in the US

The Wide Range Intelligence Test (WRIT)

The Wechsler Adult Intelligence Scale (WAIS-III)

These batteries of tests include measures of verbal comprehension, vocabulary, verbal reasoning, and working memory – to assess verbal intelligence – and measures of processing speed, non-verbal reasoning, spatial imagery, and perceptual matching – to assess non-verbal intelligence.

It has long been suggested that children with dyslexia show a characteristic profile of results on the WISC, labelled the 'ACID profile'. Four sub-tests – Arithmetic (mental arithmetic), Coding (visual short-term memory and speed of processing), Information (general knowledge and verbal comprehension), Digit span (verbal short-term memory) – are believed to be particularly difficult for dyslexic readers. More recent research, however, has shown that not all dyslexic readers show this profile, and some people who show this profile are not dyslexic.

Appendix D
Assistive technology

Text reading software
ClaroRead and ClaroRead Plus

Software that allows the individual to check text as they type. The individual highlights sections of their document and the software reads the text aloud; can also be used to read webpages or documents that the user scans into the computer. Printed text may be saved as an audio file and recorded for future listening. The colour, style, size, and spacing of the text may be quickly and easily modified. Other features include: predictive typing, identification of homophones within the document (e.g. 'there', 'their', and 'they're'), a screen ruler which can be used to magnify portions of text or change the contrast of text against background, and a talking calculator. For use with Windows Vista, XP, and 2000 (ClaroRead 2007 and ClaroRead Plus 2007); Mac OS X version 10.2.8 or later, including OSX 10.5 (ClaroRead for Mac). See www.clarosoftware.com/index.php

WordRead 2

Software that converts printed text (in Word documents, emails, pdf documents, and webpages) into human-quality speech; the user can select from seventeen languages and accents, including UK English, American English, Australian English, Swedish, Danish, Spanish, German, French, and Japanese. Printed text may be saved as an audio file and recorded for future listening. For use with

Windows 98, ME, 2000, XP, and Vista; Microsoft Word 2000, XP, 2003, and 2007. See www.clarosoftware.com/index.php

Wordbar

A bank of words created by the user that sits at the bottom of the computer screen. This may include words or phrases which the individual has the greatest difficulty spelling, and these may be sorted alphabetically or by topic. When users want to use one of the words, they click on it for it to be inserted directly into a text document, or they may hear the word spoken first by the computer (in either a standard voice or the user's own voice, once this has been recorded into the program) to ensure that they have selected the correct word. For use with Windows 95, 98, ME, NT, 2000, XP and Vista. See www.cricksoft.com/uk/default.asp

TextHELP Read&Write GOLD

Software that allows users to check text as they type into a Windows document, spreadsheet, or webpage. Includes predictive typing, a talking dictionary and thesaurus, a phonetic spellchecker, homophone checker, pronunciation tutor, and speech-enabled calculator. As the individual highlights sections of text, the software reads the text aloud in a human-quality (male or female) voice. Documents can also be scanned into the computer, or photographed with a digital camera, for the software to read. For use with Windows 2000, XP, and Vista. See www.texthelp.com/

Thunder Screen Reader (Thunder Home and Thunder Plus)

Software that 'speaks' text from Windows menus and dialog boxes, text documents, spreadsheets, and webpages (for internet access, an internet browser called WebbIE must be installed on the computer). Available in two versions – Thunder Home, which may be downloaded for free home use, and Thunder Plus, which must be purchased. Thunder Plus includes a number of extra features including the use of two human-quality voices (a British English voice and an American English voice), technical support, and voice recognition features from Dragon Naturally Speaking (see below). For use with Windows XP Home or Professional and Windows Vista. See www.screenreader.net/

AspireReader 4.0

Software that converts printed text (in rich text documents and webpages) into human-recorded or computer-generated speech; also plays digital talking books. Reading speed may be adjusted as required. For use with Windows 98, 2000, ME, and XP; Mac OS X v.10.3. See www.aequustechnologies.com/company.asp

Reading Pen

A hand-held device that can be used to scan individual words or lines of text. The text appears clearly on the display (with syllable breaks illustrated) and the device reads the words aloud with their definitions; words may also be entered into the device manually. European versions of the Pen include English (with words taken from the Concise Oxford English Dictionary), German, Swedish, and Dutch. The US version includes words from the American Heritage College Dictionary. See www.wizcomtech.com/

Textic Toolbars

Software that converts printed text into human-recorded speech at the click of a button on the toolbar. Also allows the user to change the colour, size, and font of the printed text and the background colour. Separate toolbars need to be purchased for reading text from webpages and from word documents and emails. Audio files may be saved in mp3 format for future use. For use with Windows 98, 2000, ME and XP; Mac OS10. See www.textic.com/

CapturaTalk

Software installed on a fully functional Windows Mobile Smartphone that allows users to take photographs of text wherever they are. The text is then converted to speech and saved on the phone for future reference and playback. See www.capturatalk.com/home.asp

Speech recognition software
Dragon Naturally Speaking Preferred v9

Software that allows users to create and edit text documents and emails, and to control their computer, by speaking into a micro-phone (or by playing back an audio recording from a digital voice recorder). A short period of 'training' (reading a training script into the microphone) increases the accuracy of the speech recognition software. A text-to-speech facility allows users to check the accuracy of their dictated documents. For use with Windows 2000 or higher. See www.nuance.com/

Portable recorders
Olympus DS-40 digital voice recorder

A digital voice recorder that allows the recording of up to 136 hours of audio data via a stereo microphone. Includes a voice filter and background interference reduction to maximise the quality of the recording. Audio files are stored in WMA format.

Comes with audio instructions and a clear, high-contrast, backlit LCD screen. See www.olympus-global.com/en/global/

Audio Notetaker v1.2

Software that allows the user to organise digital audio recordings (WMA, WAV, or MP3 files) by navigating through the file quickly and easily, adding notes, colour-coding sections, changing the order of sections, and editing the content of the recordings. The software presents a visual representation of the audio file, with speech and pauses shown, for easy manipulation. For use with Windows XP and Vista. See http://accessibleaudio.co.uk/

Pegasus Mobile NoteTaker

A portable hand-held device consisting of a base unit and an electronic pen (which also contains real ink) which allows the user to make hand-written notes on paper (up to A4 size), while the pen strokes (the movements of the pen) are captured by the device for later transfer directly into a computer application; built-in text recognition software allows the user's handwriting to be converted into text to be included in a word document. Up to fifty A4 sheets' worth of information (text or drawings) may be stored. For use with Microsoft Windows 2000 or XP. See www.pegatech.com/

Dyslexia-friendly fonts

Since the beginning of the twenty-first century there has been an increase in the number of specialist 'dyslexia-friendly' fonts that are available for use in webpages and books, and for individual home use. These fonts are designed to be simple, clear, and free from the additional 'ticks' and 'strokes' (the small, decorative lines) that accompany traditional 'serif' fonts. They also tend to have long ascenders (parts of the letters that rise above the midline of text, e.g. the upward strokes in the letters 'd', 'h', and 'l'), and long descenders (parts of the letters that drop below the line, e.g. the downward strokes in the letters 'g', 'j', and 'p') to make individual letters easily distinguishable.

Lexia Readable

This clear and simple font is designed to be as similar as possible to normal handwriting (with the letter 'a' represented by an 'ɑ' and a 'g' written as a 'ɡ'). Compare, for example, the following words written in Lexia (size 12):

the children enjoy reading books in school

and in the traditional Times font (also size 12):

the children enjoy reading books in school.

Lexia can be downloaded for free home use (for Mac or PC) from: www.k-type.com/fontlexia.html

Read

The design of this font began when its creator, Natascha Frensch (herself dyslexic) was a graphic design student at the Royal College of Art in London. The font is available in three versions, Read Regular (now being used by the publisher Chrysalis Books in its educational children's books), Read Smallcaps (all capital letters – see figure 15) and Read Space (a more widely spaced version for use with young children). Examples of each version of the font, and details of how to purchase it, can be found at: www.readregular.com/

FS Mencap

A font designed in collaboration with Mencap (a support organisation for people with learning disabilities), primarily for readers

Read Regular:

abcde

Read Smallcaps:

AABBCCDDEE

FS Mencap:

abcde ABCDE

Heinemann:

abcde ABCDE

Figure 15 Examples of some commercially available, dyslexia-friendly fonts

with dyslexia. The letters are designed to be clean, elegant, and easily identifiable (see figure 15). The font will be made available for individual use in the near future. Details of the font are found at: http://typophile.com/files/Mencap-Press-Pack.pdf

Heinemann Special

A family of commercially available, modern, clear fonts designed in collaboration with children, primary school teachers, special needs teachers, and dyslexic readers (figure 15 shows an example). Details of the fonts are available from: www.type.co.uk/pdfpreview/F004626.pdf

Other fonts that may be suitable for dyslexic readers include Ariel, Verdana, Geneva, Comic Sans, and Trebuchet MS, freely available with Microsoft applications, Myriad Pro (available from Adobe), and Sassoon (available from www.clubtype.co.uk/fonts/sas/sasslist_ed.html).

Mind mapping software

This enables users to create non-linear diagrams showing how pieces of information link together, and helps them to organise their ideas. This software can be useful for (1) young children, to help them to produce written stories; (2) older children, adolescents and adults, to help them to produce essays and coursework for school, college, and university; (3) adults, to help them to structure reports and presentations for work.

Claro MindFull, version 2.0

Software to aid in the development of visual concept (mind) maps. Individuals note their ideas, add images and sounds then link them together and organise them to aid the understanding of concepts during learning, the preparation of essays for assessment, and revision for exams. Concept maps may be exported directly into a Word document, a Webpage or a Powerpoint slide. For use with Windows 2000, XP and Vista. See www.clarosoftware.com/index.php

Inspiration

Software that enables individuals to produce a visual representation of linked ideas and concepts (including words, pictures, symbols, audio files, multimedia files, and hyperlinks to other documents and websites). Concepts may be organised quickly and easily within a template, and differentiated by colour, pattern, or font. At the click of a button the graphical representation (diagram view) may be converted into a hierarchical list of written ideas (outline view); both of these may be exported to word documents, webpages, and Powerpoint slides. For use with Windows 95, 98, 2000, NT 4.0, ME, XP (including Tablet PC Edition), or Vista; Mac OS 8.6, 9.x, or OS X (10.1.5 or higher). See www.inspiration.com/productinfo/inspiration/index.cfm

Kidspiration 3

Software aimed at children from kindergarten to year five, to enable them to represent their ideas in a multi-sensory way by linking pictures, symbols, text, and audio files. Children practice linking pictures together (e.g. a picture of a girl, a birthday cake, and some balloons) to tell a simple story. The words that represent the pictures (e.g. 'a girl', 'a birthday cake', 'balloons') are shown on the computer screen to help children to plan their sentences and to link these together into a story. The program incorporates a dictionary which provides for each word: (1) a textual definition; (2) a visual representation of the word's meaning; (3) a spoken pronunciation; (4) synonyms; (5) antonyms; and (6) a sample sentence including the word. Also includes visual number tasks to build mathematical awareness and spatial reasoning. For use with Windows 98, ME, 2000, XP, and Vista; Mac OS X, version 10.2.8 or newer. See www.inspiration.com/index.cfm

KidSpark

Software for children up to the age of ten years which enables them to drag and drop images (standard clipart images or their own imported images), to organise them in a visual (2-D or virtual 3-D) way, and then to link text to those images. As children manipulate the images and text, a textual representation of the 'idea map' is built up to the side of the screen. Includes a built-in text-to-speech reader. For use with Microsoft Windows 95, 98, 98SE, ME, NT, 2000, or XP; Mac OS X 10.2 or 10.3. See www.spark-space.com/products.htm

Mind genius (Home Edition, Education, Business)

Mind mapping software for the home, for schools, and for businesses. Each version is designed to facilitate the organisation of concepts in a visual way; maps may then be exported into Word documents, pdf documents, webpages, or PowerPoint presentations. For use with Windows 98, 2000, Millenium edition, Vista, and XP. See www.mindgenius.com

MindManager

Software designed to allow users to organise and communicate ideas visually, to plan projects in detail, and to demonstrate the relationships between individual concepts. Maps may be exported as images or in text format to Microsoft Office applications, pdf documents, and webpages. For use with Windows Vista and XP (MindManager Pro 7); Mac OS X 10.4.x and OS X 10.5.x (MindManager 7 Mac). See www.mindjet.com

Training software

Clicker 5

A computer program to help young children to construct sentences without using the keyboard by selecting words and phrases from the lower half of the screen. The child clicks on the word or phrase and the computer 'speaks' it; if the child is happy with the word/phrase that he/she has selected, it can be added to his/her sentence at the top of the screen. The expanding sentence can be read back to the child with each word being highlighted as it is spoken. For use with Windows 98, ME, NT, 2000, XP, and Vista; Mac OS X 10.3 or higher. See www.cricksoft.com/uk/default.asp

PC How To IT training software

A collection of over 70,000 online tutorials (each lasting approx-imately two minutes) to teach the user various IT skills (includ-ing instruction in the use of Word, Excel, PowerPoint, Outlook, Visio, Lotus Notes, and others) without the need to read technical instruction manuals. Beginner, Intermediate, and Advanced level instruction is available for each application. For use with Windows 95, 98, NT 4.0 Service Pack 3, or higher. See www.pchowto.com/ or www.pchowtouk.com/

Aspire Video Based learning Tool

A CD-ROM-based collection of seventy-three videos (over an hour in total) to teach students study skills strategies relating to research, composition, note-taking, proofreading, and time-management. Includes instruction in the use of Microsoft Office and Windows Vista as well as the use of assistive technology products (e.g. Dragon Naturally Speaking, MindManager, and ClaroRead). See www.claroreadxtras.com/

Nessy Brain Booster

Software designed for teenagers and adults to help them to develop independent study skills. As the individual explores the different sections (covering reading skills, writing skills, organi-sational skills, revision skills, and memory skills) they view visual images and simple animations, try interactive activities, and read text (with text-to-speech software) to teach them strategies to support their learning. For use with Windows 98 or later. See www.nessy.co.uk/

Englishtype Junior and Englishtype Senior

Teach yourself touch typing programs for children aged seven to twelve years (Englishtype Junior) and for children and adults from the age of thirteen years (Englishtype Senior). Includes spoken and written instructions with a strong visual component (large, simple visual images with bold colours) to enhance the multi-sensory approach. Individuals follow short, self-contained lessons and are motivated as they progress. Typing proficiency may be obtained within a week. For use with Windows 98 or later. See www.englishtype.com/Englishtype.htm

KAZ Home User Typing Tutor

Teach yourself touch typing for ages five years to adult. Available in a range of options for different ages including First Keys to Literacy; KAZ Primary School Typing Tutor; KAZ Secondary School Typing Tutor; KAZ FE/HE Education Typing Tutor; and KAZ Home User Typing Tutor, each with age-appropriate instruction, words, and phrases. For use with Windows 95 or later; Mac OS 8.1 or later. See www.kaz-type.com/

Type to Learn

A touch typing ('keyboard skills') course for individuals from grade three to adult. Consists of twenty-five multi-sensory lessons and games that also teach phonics-based spelling, grammar, punctuation, composition, and dictation skills. For use with Windows 95 or later; Mac OS7.0 or later (excluding OSX). See http://store.sunburst.com/

Dictionaries

Franklin DMQ-1870 Electronic dictionary

A hand-held, portable dictionary, thesaurus, and phonetic spell checker (e.g. identifies the word 'nite' as 'night'). Contains over half a million words from the Collins Concise Dictionary, as well as the entire Collins Concise Thesaurus; also includes idioms, specialist legal, medical, business, and engineering terms, and crossword and anagram solvers. See www.franklin-uk. co.uk/ or www.franklin.com/

Franklin Talking Dictionaries

A range of hand-held electronic dictionaries, with features including word meanings, pronunciation guides, word usage guidelines, spellings for phonetically entered words, idioms, quotations, thesaurus, and grammar guides. All of these dictionaries come with text-to-speech capability. Within the range of devices are dictionaries designed for individuals of different ages (children and adults) and educational levels, including the following:

- Children's Talking Dictionary & Spell Corrector;
- Merriam-Webster Speaking Dictionary & Thesaurus;
- Merriam-Webster's Speaking Executive Dictionary with Thesaurus;
- Speaking Merriam-Webster's Collegiate Dictionary, 11th Edition
- Speaking Merriam-Webster's Collegiate Dictionary, 11th Edition with Deluxe 5-Language Suite
- Speaking Collins English Dictionary & Thesaurus with Advanced English Reference Suite;
- Speaking Language Master;
- Speaking Language Master Special Edition
  See www.franklin.com/

Memory aids

Timely Reminders

Freeware that may be downloaded onto a PC and used to facilitate independent learning by children or adults. Questions and answers on any topic of study may be entered into the software (visual images and audio files may also be included) for the individual to attempt as many times, and as regularly, as they feel is necessary until the information has been learned. The same questions may be presented for example every day, every two days, every week, every month, or so on. For use with Windows 95, 98, 2000, NT4. See www.timelyreminders. co.uk/

Mastering Memory

Software designed to enable individuals (child or adult) to develop their visual and auditory memory through a series of tasks involving the presentation of age-appropriate pictures, written words, signs and symbols, and/or spoken words. Through remembering and recalling lists of items the individual may develop effective visual and auditory memory strategies. For use with Windows 2000, NT4, XP, and Vista. See www. masteringmemory.co.uk/

Memory booster

Software to help develop children's visual and verbal memory skills through playing an adventure game of increasing difficulty. Designed for children aged four to eleven years. For use with Windows 98, ME, 2000, and XP. See www.memory-booster. com/

Colour screening and visual aids

Intuitive Colorimeter System

This device determines whether an individual can benefit from the use of coloured lenses during reading. Text is viewed through a window while the colour of the ambient light in the device may be altered in terms of its hue (colour), saturation (strength of colour), and luminance (brightness). The individual decides which colour, if any, best helps to eliminate the visual distortions that they experience while reading. For a list of specialists around the world who provide testing on the Intuitive Colorimeter System, see www.ceriumvistech.co.uk/Specialists.htm

Coloured overlay screener

A computer program in which individuals view text presented against different-coloured backgrounds to allow them to decide which coloured background best reduces visual discomfort during reading. The results of this five-minute test identify the colour of overlay that best suits the individual; his/her computer screen may also be set to this same colour. See www.ioosales.co.uk/

Coloured overlays

A4-size coloured overlays that are placed over pages of text to reduce visual distortion and glare. Overlays are available in a range of colours that may be used alone or in combination to produce the colour best suited to the individual. See www.ioosales.co.uk, www.crossboweducation.com/ and www.ceriumvistech.co.uk/Overlays.htm

Crossbow reading rulers

Strips of narrow coloured plastic, similar to the A4 overlays, that are placed over lines of printed text; these strips are more convenient and discrete than the full size overlays. Available from www.crossboweducation.com/

Tinted glasses

Increasing numbers of optical practitioners are now prescribing glasses with tinted lenses following testing with coloured overlays and filters to determine the most suitable colour. For a list of specialists around the world who dispense glasses with coloured lenses see www.eyecare-trust.org.uk or http://irlen. com/clinicfinder.php

ReadAble

Software that enables the user to customise the colour and font of the computer desktop and the settings of Windows applications, including the background colour, text colours, toolbars, font size, style, and spacing. These changes may be made automatically by pressing the ReadAble icon on the computer. For use with Windows 2000 and XP. See www.dyslexic.com/

ClaroView

Software that may be used to change the colour and tint (brightness) of the computer screen. For use with Windows 2000, XP, and Vista. See www.clarosoftware. com/

Optim-Eyes Reading Lamps

Desk lamps that enable users to alter the colour of the ambient lighting (by adjusting sixty red, green, and blue LEDs), to find the colour of light that best suits their needs. Designed to reduce visual stress and glare. See www.dyslexic.com/

Appendix E
Websites

The following websites are good sources of information on dyslexia:

The homepage of 'amidyslexic?com' for online dyslexia screening
www.amidyslexic.com/

The homepage of the British Dyslexia Centre
www.britishdyslexiacentre.com/bdc/homedefault.aspx

The information and resource download page of Dyslexia High Peak
www.d-hp.co.uk/downloads.html

The homepage of Dyslexia International – Tools & Technologies
www.ditt-online.org/About.htm

The homepage of 'Dyslexia Help'
www.dyslexiahelp.co.uk/index.html

The homepage of 'the World Of Dyslexia' with resources for (1) parents of dyslexic children; (2) dyslexic adults; and (3) dyslexic students at college or university
www.dyslexia-parent.com
www.dyslexia-adults.com
www.dyslexia-college.com/index.htm

The homepage of the Dyslexia Research Trust
  www.dyslexic.org.uk

The homepage of LD (learning difficulties) Online
  www.ldonline.org

The homepage of Listening Books – The National Listening
Library (UK)
  www.listening-books.org.uk

The homepage of RFB&D (Recording for the Blind &
Dyslexic) for audio books (USA)
  www.rfbd.org

The homepage of PATOSS (the Professional Association of
Teachers of Students with Specific learning difficulties)
  www.patoss-dyslexia.org/index.html

Index

Page numbers in *italics* refer to illustrations